Back Off! I'll lose weight when I'm ready.

The ultimate weight loss guide for teens and their crazed parents!

- Why dieting makes weight loss harder
- How to eat at school
- Controlling eating disorders
- Smoking & weight management
- Easy tips for faster weight loss

By Debi Davis

Published by Frederick Fell Publishers, Inc.
www.fellpub.com

Davis, Debi.
  Back off! : I'll lose weight when I'm ready : the ultimate weight loss guide for teens and their crazed parents! / by Debi Davis.
      p. cm.
  ISBN 0-88391-104-3 (pbk. : alk. paper)
  1. Obesity in adolescence. 2. Weight loss. 3. Obesity in adolescence--
Psychological aspects. 4. Body image in adolescence. I. Title.
  RJ399.C6D385 2004
  613.2'5--dc22

                                        2004003165

Cover/Interior Design by Chris Hetzer
Printed in USA

10 9 8 7 6 5 4 3 2 1

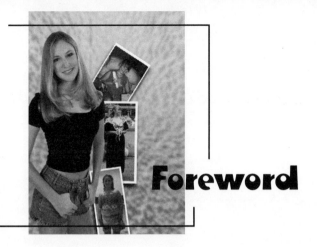

Foreword

My name is Blake Davis. I was fat. Actually, I was born fat. I came into this world at 10-1/2 pounds and kept growing! My mom wrote this book. In 1997, when I was twelve, I was 26 pounds overweight and hated the way I looked. I used to sneak chips and candy home from school and hide them under my bed and in my drawers so I could snack when no one was watching. I even stopped eating altogether when I really felt guilty about what I ate.

Having a mom in the weight loss business wasn't an advantage in my house. I already was unhappy that my parents got divorced. Staying fat was my way of teaching them both a lesson. But, I found that I was the one that really learned something: My parents got along great once they didn't live together anymore and were both happy with their lives. Unfortunately, I was pretty unhappy with mine.

Once I decided to make a few changes, it didn't take long for me to lose the extra 26 pounds. Now that I know what to eat, it's been really easy for me to keep the weight off and not gain it back. I've stayed in shape since 1998 and I'm pretty proud of myself for taking control. I like the way I look now a lot better than when I was heavy, too.

Everything in this book is what I learned along the way. I know it will help you if you really want to lose weight. It's up to you. No one can lose weight for you.

Just stick to your plan and keep visualizing your picture and you'll do great.

Good luck,

Blake

So...You Think You Have a Weight Problem?

Congratulations, you've made the first step. You recognize that you're not satisfied with the way you look and you've already done something about it: You're reading this book! There is no question that just by reading this book you won't suddenly be in shape like Cameron Diaz or Leonardo de Caprio, but you will find that you can control how you look and how you feel. It's just a matter of how important it is to you to make the necessary changes in order to do so.

First, let me tell you, your weight problem is most likely not your fault. There are a zillion reasons why people are overweight and they don't necessarily have to do with food. Now hold on...I'm not suggesting that a lot of the junk you probably eat and certainly don't need, doesn't contribute to your problem. The fact is, when you better understand yourself and learn how to select smart foods, then losing weight becomes 'a piece of cake' so to speak.

Here's the deal. Weight problems are 50% physical and 50% psychological. The physical part is obvious. The psychological side is a little more complicated. What we're going to do in this book is take a look at all aspects of what makes you tick (and eat!) and let you find your own solutions...realistic solutions that you can live with comfortably.

The first step is to be honest with yourself. You cannot change any habits, good or bad, if you don't acknowledge that these habits exist. Likewise, you can't stop feeding a sweet tooth if you deny that you overindulge in sweets. I, myself, had a cheese and sweets problem. I sort of knew about the sweets part. If I found myself in a stressful or upsetting situation, the only comfort I could supply myself with was chocolate...Anything chocolate! I think I could have probably eaten a shoe if it was dipped and chocolate-coated like a Dove Bar. Fortunately, I was very aware that sweets and stress went hand-in-hand for me. Knowing this helped when I wanted to lose weight. Recognizing my personal need for some form of comfort in a stressful situation, I needed to find myself a reward that wouldn't pack additional pounds on my butt.

This is not a diet book. I'm not going ask you to diet because diets don't work. Sure, you'll lose a little weight - maybe even a lot. But most diets require eliminating things you love to eat or planning everything you put into your mouth every day, and that's not realistic. We're going to make it simple and do it together. Once you better understand what foods actually help you lose and what makes you gain, it will be really easy for you to eat smart and stay fit. And let's face facts, puking isn't pretty and it wouldn't make you the hit of any party if everyone knew what you were doing (which they probably do) so don't even think about purging to stay in shape. Not only are you screwing up your entire body's system by making it impossible to process food adequately, it could kill you.

You may find some items I discuss to be duplicated from section to section. That's because the information I'm providing is important and needs to be addressed as it applies to various topics throughout this book.

If you're getting grief from your parents or friends about how you eat or the fact that you're 'expanding' a little, tell them (politely) to "Back Off" and show them my message at the end of this book. If they continue to give you a hard time, have them call me. No kidding. I'd be happy to speak with them because you and I are in this together.

Weight loss success is about commitment. You need to be committed to making a change in how you look, what you eat and how you feel. I may tell you to eat more and you're going to have to trust me. I lost 85 pounds. My daughter lost 26 pounds when she was only 12. You think you've got a problem? Try having a mom in the weight loss business when you're a 12-year-old wearing a ladies' size 13!

You're going to do great. Take a deep breath. Make a picture in your mind of the way you want to look. (Don't mess with me and create a picture that includes your sprouting up to 5'11 when your entire family is no taller than 5'5!) See yourself slim & trim. Let yourself imagine how great you're going to feel when you reach your weight goal. This is not just play imagery, you know. You can really accomplish this if you set your mind to it. It's not hard. It just takes a little patience and perseverance. You didn't gain your weight overnight. You won't lose it overnight either. But you're going to feel so much better every step of the way.

Good luck!

Debi Davis

TABLE OF CONTENTS

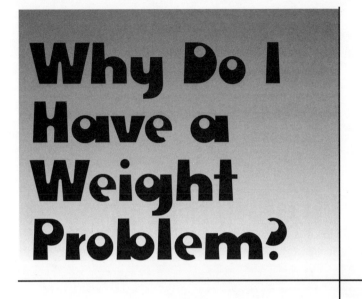

chapter one

Why Do I Have a Weight Problem?

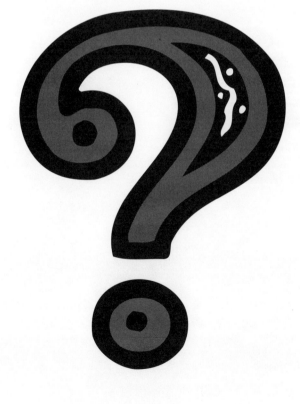

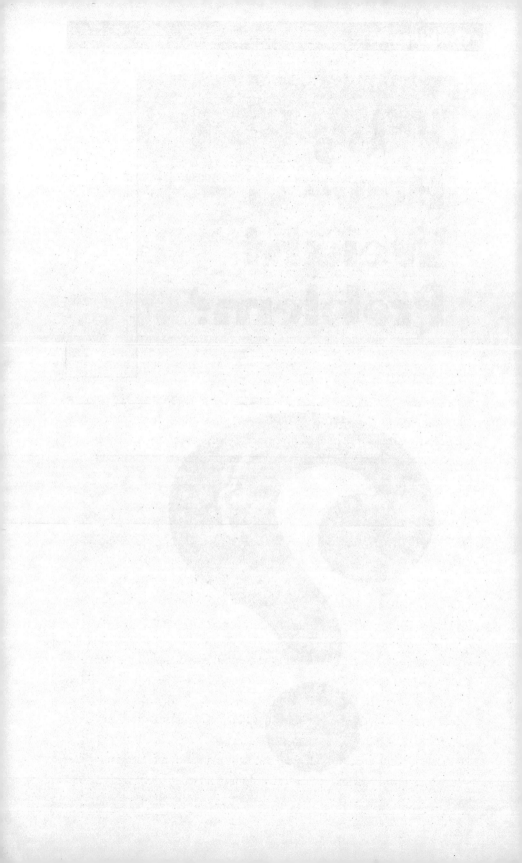

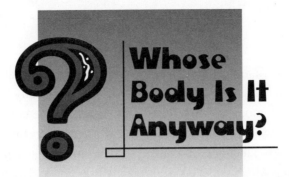

Whose Body Is It Anyway?

If you think you could lose a few pounds or would feel much better in smaller jeans, you're in luck. Once you understand how your brain and body works, it will be much easier to make smart food choices and proceed down the path to personal fitness.

First of all, think of your body as a machine. It generally runs at a consistent pace and processes whatever you provide it in the form of nutrition through the food you eat. Metabolism is a term used to describe the activity and speed in which your body processes food. When your metabolism is slow, it is much easier for you to gain weight. If it is fast, you may need to eat high calorie food supplements to keep from becoming too thin.

There are a lot of things that can cause your metabolism to slow down. A change in exercise or activity patterns, excessive dieting, nutrition or hormone imbalances, having children, all contribute to a slowing of your metabolic level.

Think of your body like a machine that requires maintenance just like a car. If you drive, you are aware your car needs gas in order for it to go. Likewise, when you change your oil, the mechanic usually also changes the oil filter. This enables the car to run cleaner and more efficiently, which reduces your gas consumption. Your body is no different. It needs gas (or in this case, food) to operate. And, eating a different selection of foods every day helps the body process that food more efficiently so your body runs cleaner...just like with a clean oil filter.

Eating the same food all the time will cause toxins to form. When you rotate your food and eat different items every day, your body will get rid of the old food first. Let me give you a better example of what I mean. If chicken is something you eat just about every day, your body will have a hard time figuring out which is today's chicken from the chicken you ate yesterday or the day before. If 3-day old chicken remains in your body, (is that a gross thought, or what!) you have a much greater chance of toxins forming which will slow your metabolism down even further.

Confused? Don't be. What's important, is for you to understand that just by rotating your foods and eating something different every day, you can help keep your body running at a much higher performance level.

Not taking control of yourself and the food you eat is certainly NOT one of your options. If you're not proud of the way you look or find yourself avoiding friendships because you don't feel like you 'fit in', do something about it! If you continue to let food control you and stay heavier than you should, you run the risk of an alarming number of medical conditions that are directly related to weight such as heart disease, osteoarthritis, hypertension, diabetes and even stroke. Don't think these things can't happen to young people. It happens all the time. But it's NOT going to happen to YOU! Information is a wonderful thing...use it!

Taking control of your life is a life-changing decision that will have positive benefits for you forever. At this stage, your body and getting a good education are really the only things that you can take charge of because both of these things are directly associated with you. Every action we take affects another. If you eat poorly, your health and body will show the results. If you eat right, you feel great, look great and have tons of energy. If you study poorly and don't show interest in your schoolwork, your grades will show the result. But, when you eat right, you give your body the 'brain food' it needs to stay smart and focused on the tasks at hand. It's really that simple.

You may as well learn now that there are consequences to just about everything we do. Good consequences and bad ones. Fortunately, we can be responsible for most of the possible consequences because we control ourselves. Now that you have decided that you want to look great and feel great, you need to do the things required for the consequence of good health to be your outcome. And, is it ever worth it!

Understand the Facts and Lose the Excuses

As serious as it may seem, don't take life too seriously. In a world that may seem full of confusion and somewhat out of control, the one thing you can take charge of is yourself. Looking and feeling great is a lot easier than you probably think. The biggest step you need to take is to decide YOU want to see a change in your body. It's not enough if you're doing it because your family or friends are encouraging you. Getting in shape is YOUR decision. YOU are the one who ultimately decides what you put in your mouth so YOU need to be the one to decide to take control.

Don't beat yourself up for having gotten heavier than you should have in the first place. Most likely, you haven't done anything wrong. You probably eat pretty well and have become a victim of food misinformation like some of the adults in your life. If you're too hard on yourself, you'll get depressed or frustrated and the next thing you know, you'll be reaching for Oreo Double Stuffs to make you feel better. So, STOP IT NOW!

It's important to understand that TV and news media constantly tell us that eating "high volume, low-fat food" (which are starches like potatoes, rice, bread and pasta) are fat-free and, therefore, the best food choices you can make. Not true. Eating a lot of starch can turn your body into a fat-manufacturing machine! Carbohydrates and starches are your body's energy sources. They turn themselves into sugar to create more energy for you. If you are not exercising, your body can't possibly use all the sugar created by eating high-carbohydrate food and will turn the unused sugar into fat. When you understand that it takes 15 minutes of jogging for your body to burn off one slice of low-calorie bread, you can see how you'll need to limit the starches you eat in order to lose weight.

Just for the record, I want you to be aware that there are three things that can happen to the calories you consume:

1. They can be used to meet the energy needs of the body;

2. They can be stored away as white fat (not a pretty picture);

3. They can be burned up by special cells in the body known as "brown adipose tissue," or BAT. This last "BAT" thing is really called "thermogenesis," meaning the generation of heat or 'burning up calories,' and is a normal body process similar to digestion.

The purpose of BAT (or thermogenesis) is to burn up the calories your body doesn't need. Being overweight, or obese, occurs primarily when BAT is not working right and you have a very slow metabolism, so the body must deal with excess calories by storing them as fat.

Under the right circumstances, the body may even convert stored calories back into the kind of calories that can be gotten rid of through 'thermal combustion,' which is a fancy way of saying fat burn. Fat burn is your body's way of using the food you eat. This process serves two critical functions. First, it prevents the fat in your body that hasn't been permanently attached to you yet from being stored on you in areas such as tummy, hips and thighs. And, second, it converts or breaks down the current stored fat that's already stuck on you somewhere into fat that may be burned off.

For many years, scientists have been trying to discover what goes wrong with the thermogenic process. Why do some people stay thin by burning off excess calories, yet other people seem to be unable to do this and put on extra pounds and inches instead? Sound familiar??? Consider, for example, something you may have to look forward to: "middle-age spread." That's when your tummy or butt just seems to get bigger for no good reason as you get older.

Scientists figure that the sudden weight gain many people between the ages of 30 and 40 experience may be the result of the shut down of the BAT (or thermogenic) process. They think that something genetic may be the reason. If your parents or grandparents are heavy, it is possible that you have inherited that same genetic link to being overweight, so check out your family tree. If the branches seem to be hanging really, really low... LOOK OUT!

One thing I can tell you from personal experience is that even after losing 85 pounds, I still consider myself to be a fat person in a thin suit. I came from a family of 'overeaters' that were always on one diet or another. So, I guess what I'm really telling you is that you can break this cycle just like I did. It just means that you may have to work a little harder at it than other people do with your same weight problem if being overweight tends to run in your family.

I hate to say it, but it's pretty clear that most school systems today have limited time for physical education and their cafeterias feature high-carbohydrate foods like pasta, pizza, and burgers. When you think about it, you have actually been educated to have weight problems so...it's time to fight back! I can't wait for you to experience how great it feels when you turn down the pizza and reach for the chicken breast instead. Doing the right thing for your body can make you feel so terrific. It also reinforces the fact that YOU are in control of YOU!

I want to share a few interesting statistics with you so you can better understand how common it is for young people to be fighting against obesity:

• The city and state where you live can play a part in your chances to be overweight. According to a report from the Centers of Disease Control and Prevention, children living in New York, for example, are 'substantially more overweight' than children living elsewhere in the country. Overall, almost 20% of New York's third-graders and over 21% of sixth-graders are overweight. The national statistics for other parts of the country show, on average, that 12.5 - 14.7% of boys & girls aged 6 to 11 are overweight.

Now, get real for a minute...after looking at statistics like these, do you think you can expect to be automatically thin as a teenager when the chances are great that you have been conditioned to being overweight from as young as 5 or 6 year old?

Here are some more...

• More than 97-MILLION people in the U.S. are obese, which means that the amount of fat on their body accounts for more than 25% of their weight for men and 30%for women. More than 50% of Americans feel they need to lose weight. Thirty-billion dollars per year is spent on weight-reduction programs and special foods that encourage weight loss or weight management.

• Ethnic cultures make a significant difference, too.   Different religious or ethnic groups tend to focus on different types of foods that historically have been part of their heritage regardless if those foods are good for them or not.Mexican-Americans eat a lot of beans, rice and casserole-type combinations. African-Americans prefer frying food as their method of cooking.

Here's the real deal: If weight problems run in your family, that certainly contributes to your present weight level as well. Obesity tends to run in families but it's not always caused by the genes you were born with. (Please notice I said genes and not "jeans!") Sometimes it's a physical thing - most often, it's poor food awareness and over-indulgence (that means you eat too often or too much of the wrong stuff!).

Before you get too far down the road with any weight loss program, make sure your family doctor has checked you for any one of a number of rare illnesses that can cause obesity. Hypothyroidism, Depression, Cushing's syndrome, as well as reactions to a variety of drugs like steroids or antidepressants may cause weight gain.

I know I don't need to remind you that being overweight is a definite health hazard. People who let their weight get out of control and are more than forty percent overweight for ten years or more are twice as likely to die prematurely than a person of average weight. Not to mention all the serious medical conditions that obesity can cause. In fact, obesity has even been associated with higher rates of certain types of cancer in both men and women. I don't want to scare you, but you need to know what can happen if you don't decide to get a grip on your eating now.

If your family is like most families in America, you share the same diet and lifestyle habits as your mom, dad and your brothers & sisters, which contributes to an overweight condition for everybody. Taste and/or convenience are not the best reason for selecting the foods you eat. I can tell you one thing, if you get your weight under control now and learn to eat right, it's highly unlikely that you will have a weight problem when you hit adulthood. Most of the kids I've worked with have lost their weight and kept it off better than their parents. In most cases, the kids started giving their parents grief about what they ate. It was like the kids became the parents because they were more aware of what was good for them than their elders! See what you have to look forward to!

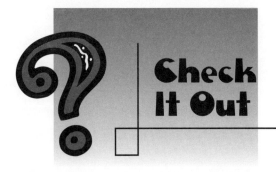

Check It Out

Every bit of the information in this book is going to help you take control of YOU. But, there are lots of factors that can contribute to an overweight condition in young people. You'll want to rule out any physical problems before you frustrate yourself further by trying to make your body do something it's physically unable to do. If you think you eat pretty well and your weight problem doesn't make much sense, go see your doctor and have him give you a check up.

The thyroid gland, which is near the throat and regulates your growth can be responsible for all kinds of weight complications. Having an under-active or over-active thyroid can cause weight gain. Food sensitivities or food allergies are two conditions that cause the body to react negatively to proper food processing or fat elimination.

You may be hypo or hyper-glycemic, which is a super-high or super-low amount of sugar in the blood. Either of these conditions can cause you to eat constantly throughout the day. Another possibility is diabetes. Diabetes, (a condition that causes elevated blood sugar), may cause you to experience sugar cravings that you have always just figured to be because of an "out of control sweet tooth."

Or, you may be in perfect health and just need to re-evaluate your eating and lifestyle habits. Let's just be sure. See your doctor and have him check you for all the various conditions that may aggravate or cause an overweight condition so you really know exactly what your body is dealing with.

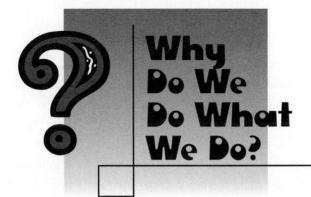

Why Do We Do What We Do?

Before you can get a handle on all of the changes that you want to make to better yourself, let's first go over how your brain works along with some of the things you may need to understand in order for you to make changes easily.

Your brain has two sides. One side is the logical side. The other is the emotional side. The logical side is the side where you learn things and deal with issues from a real and factual point of view. It's the same side of your brain that helps you figure out what's right from wrong and what's good from bad.

The emotional side of your brain is the side that creates reactions or responses to things that happen to you throughout the day. If someone says something mean to you at school, you may feel angry, sad or defensive. These are all emotional responses. Some people act more aggressively than others when they respond to things around them. An automatic emotional response for an out-of-control-type person may be to hit anybody who gives them trouble or gets in their way. Know anybody like that?

Everyones' responses are personal. They are also learned and do not come naturally all by themselves. Emotional responses are automatic responses that come from unconscious thought. Logical responses are those you are conscious or fully aware of making.

From the time we are babies, we learn to respond to things that happen around us. Think of the emotional side of your brain as having a giant filing cabinet attached to it. In that filing cabinet are all of the emotional responses we have collected from the very beginning of our life.

When something happens to make us happy, we file that memory away. We do the same thing if something upsets us. We immediately go into our emotional filing cabinet to see how we should react and file that action away, too.

The emotional side of your brain will override the logical side of your brain every time unless you consciously stop it. If you are at a great party, and it's getting close to your curfew time, the emotional side of your brain may say, "I'm having a great time and I don't want to go home." The logical side says, "You need to go home - that is the rule." Your emotional side says, "I don't care about rules, I'm having fun." Then, the logical side steps in once more to remind you that... "If I don't go home on time, my parents will yell at me and get me all upset. Then they will probably ground me for the rest of the week which would be beyond awful. Staying out isn't worth the emotional nightmare it will create for me. I guess I'll leave the party and go home." The logical side of your brain, when used, can help the emotional side see reason, so let yourself at least hear what it has to say.

Smoking is a great example of emotions overriding logic. I hope this example does not apply to you because I would hate to think that you smoke, especially knowing all the hazards, but, I am sure you know someone who does. Logically, a smoker is fully aware that they are jeopardizing their health by smoking. But, emotionally, the comfort they attach to smoking is more important to them and the danger of the activity no longer matters.

Everyone starts to smoke for a reason. That reason is attached to some sort of emotion that they have filed away in their emotional filing cabinet. Someone may smoke because it makes them feel sophisticated, more grown up, sexy, rebellious or because their friends all do it and they want to fit in. None of these are really great reasons to screw up your lungs or other parts of your body, but they may be just the reasons the young smoker uses to justify their decision to partake in a really disgusting and stinky habit.

What you are doing right now by reading this book is starting to build up the tools you'll need to take control and plan your life logically. When you let the logical side of your brain take over, you'll find you'll almost always make the right decision. Today you may be living your life solely from the emotional side of your brain, which can be very dangerous. Depending upon what's in all the emotional files you've collected up until this point, the emotional side of your brain might be full of all the wrong reactions...like overeating in times of stress.

Well, we're going to fix that. As of this moment, you're the boss. You're in charge of YOU and you can do anything you set your mind to. So, let's learn a little more...

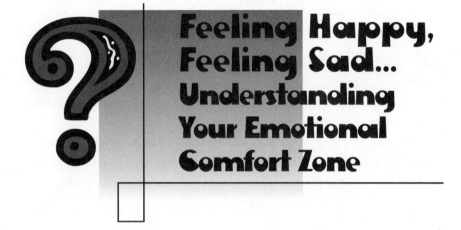

Feeling Happy, Feeling Sad... Understanding Your Emotional Comfort Zone

Now that you have a better understanding of how your brain works, let's move to the next level so you can further understand what makes us do the things we do. In addition to the two sides of our brain, all of us have an invisible emotional median that serves as a dividing line between positive and negative or good and bad feelings. The brain's goal is to try and keep us as emotionally positive and happy as possible. Our emotions will let us sit right on the median because that is an acceptable comfort zone. But, our emotions usually try to keep our happiness level a little above it. When something happens to upset us and we are unhappy or feel insecure, that's when our emotions fall below the median line. Our brain will then immediately dip into our emotional filing cabinet to find the fastest way to get our emotions back up above the median line so we can feel happy again.

ABOVE THE LINE: confidence
                             happiness
                             contentment
                             bliss

_____emotional median - acceptable comfort zone_____

                             insecurity
                             sadness
                             fear
BELOW THE LINE: frustration

When we live "above the line" on our emotional median we are happy and content. But, on the other hand, if something happens that takes us into an upsetting condition and drops our emotions "below the line," we immediately look to the emotional side of our brain to tell us what to do in order to feel better.

Using the smoking example from the last section, I want to illustrate how the building of our emotional files work and how long the file stays with us even though the original idea for the file may not even make any sense for us anymore.

At the time a smoker takes their first cigarette, there is an emotion that they feel which encourages them to continue smoking. As I said before, for teens, smoking may make them feel older and more sophisticated. Soon their confidence may even be tied to their smoking habit - "When I smoke, I'm cool." For some, their reason for smoking may be because it's the least of all the pressures put on them by their peers. They may want to fit in but don't want to go so far as to do drugs or drink.

Whatever the emotional reasons are for smoking, they are neatly filed into several emotional files, one for each of the feelings that smoking generates for them.

In my example here, the act of smoking would now fall into four files:

- feeling older
- feeling more sophisticated
- feeling confident or cool
- fitting in with friends

When a situation arises that takes your emotions below-the-line and causes you to feel insecure, the emotional side of the brain goes into your: "I need to feel confident file," and suggests all of your action options that will make you feel better fast. In a split second, your brain will find the one that will provide relief the quickest - the one that can be done automatically and without conscious thought. The smoker knows that they can have a cigarette to feel more confident - more in control, so they light up because that was the file that the emotional side of their brain used.

Obviously, having the cigarette only made the smoker feel more confident because that is part of their historical belief and emotional filing system. 'Lighting up' certainly did nothing to actually improve their real confidence level. But, your beliefs create your reality. The smoker believed that a cigarette would help make an uncomfortable situation more comfortable, and therefore, it did. The fact that whatever upset them or caused their emotions to fall below-the-line in the first place, still needs to be faced. Somehow, with a cigarette, the smoker feels more able to cope with the situation. Smoking seems pretty dumb when you look at it this way, doesn't it?

The same pattern could be happening to you with food. For a lot of people, food is very comforting when they are upset. If you have a bad day at school, a candy bar or a pizza may be just the thing to make you feel better right away. It may give you an immediate emotional lift to take your emotions "above-the-line." But later, that candy bar or pizza will probably be a source of guilt for you and send you on another emotional roller-coaster, taking you even further below-the-line than you were before.

The only way to deal with a problem is to face it, evaluate it and solve it. Hiding it behind food or any other source of false comfort doesn't make the problem go away, it only makes you feel less in control. The best part is, when you actually meet the challenge head on, you feel strong, capable and really proud of yourself! Each and every time you have a success by overcoming an obstacle that you'd really rather avoid, you're building up your emotional filing cabinet with positive and empowering solutions that you can draw on later when a similar challenge comes your way.

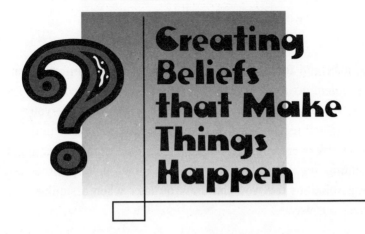

Creating Beliefs that Make Things Happen

I bet you had no idea how powerful your mind was in controlling your body. Well, the fact is, your personal reality, which is the way you live your life, is what your mind says it is. Your reality is made up from a series of personal beliefs that have developed over a period of time with the help of friends, family and personal experience. What you <u>think</u> actually determines how you act and how your body feels. If you think you are smart, you will act smart. If you think you can be successful at overcoming your weight problems, you can.

A belief will stay a belief until you change your mind and decide to believe something different. YOU have complete control over your belief system even if that belief system is greatly influenced by your parents, teachers and friends. What you do with what you learn is up to you. You can use your beliefs to create both positive or negative situations in your life. YOU control YOU.

Using the 'smart' example, let me explain a little bit more about how this idea actually works. If you think you're smart, you will use all of the information that comes out of your emotional files that you have built up over the years since you've been in school. You will use the files that tell you to: "Do your homework and pay attention in class or else you'll get in trouble." By doing what your files tell you to do, you will ultimately promote your own ability to actually BE smart. This belief system can work in a positive or negative way. For example, if you think you are shy, you will be shy when you meet people because your belief system says so, and your emotional file system supports that belief. If you think you are able to be successful in what you set out to do, you will be, if that's what you truly believe. Your fate in life is directly connected with your commitment to your beliefs. If you want to lose weight and feel better about yourself, you can do it. But first, YOU must BELIEVE that you can do it.

Don't let anyone tell you that you are unable to be an achiever. You can be whomever you want to be... It's entirely up to you. It may take work on your part to reach all the goals you'd like to set for yourself, but getting there is all about your desire and your willingness to take responsibility for your own actions. You want to lose weight and be more attractive? You can. You can do anything.

You can make the choices that best fit your needs, dreams and desires. You can make the choice to be healthy, change your appearance and lose weight. Or not. You can even make the choice to be happy. You may ultimately decide that you are happy with the way you look and choose to do nothing about the extra pounds you are carrying around. It's all up to you.

Ready to take on the challenge?

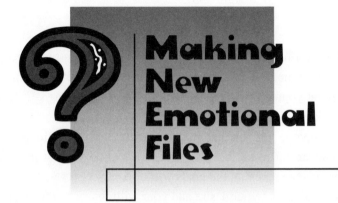

Making New Emotional Files

Now that I've got you really thinking, don't feel upset about some of the emotional responses that you know you may already have that you feel may be working against you? If we can identify the behaviors that cause you to overeat or eat the wrong things, all we need to do is clean out your old response files and replace them with better responses. Once we do that, you will find yourself a lot happier and much more in control of all your actions. This is not a big deal if you're a willing 'housekeeper!'

Think about it, you have been taught or "programmed" by your parents to act a certain way since you were a baby. A lot of those reactions have been associated in some way with food. When you cried, you got a bottle. When you were good, you got a cookie. If you finished everything on your plate, you could have dessert. Look at the emotional files that were created for you before you even knew how to create them! Even fast food restaurants like McDonald's and Burger King encourage you to feel rewarded for eating poorly. They give you "Happy Meals" that come complete with toys. Think about it. You are actually rewarded for eating a fatty cheeseburger, fries and sugary coke with a dumb toy you probably lost in the car before you ever even got home! I have run across a lot of kids and adults that have eaten high-fat fast-food for so long, they don't even like the taste of healthy meals any more. Isn't that sad?

If you turn to food at times of stress or for comfort in any way, these patterns can be changed too but, first you must face the fact that these patterns exist. Once you truly believe that you are absolutely capable of changing bad habits, the rest is pretty easy. Sometimes, all it takes is knowing what the better options are and that is what this book is all about.

Remember, a belief is a belief until you change your mind and decide to believe something else. For the best weight loss results, food should be part of your belief system in three areas only:

- I need food for my body to operate efficiently.
- Good nutrition is better for me.
- Eating properly makes me feel good.

I hope you've noticed that I have not associated food as an emotional support option. Food is a fuel supply for your body only. That doesn't mean that you can't enjoy eating or find eating out with friends to be really fun, it only means that food is not part of your emotional response files. Food's only purpose is to keep you healthy and nourished. You need to reprogram any beliefs you may have that:

- Food is a source of comfort.
- Food makes me happy.
- Food is a reward.

Let your emotions be supported with actions and not with things that you put in your mouth like food, alcohol or drugs. These items don't solve problems, they will just create more problems for you in the very near future.

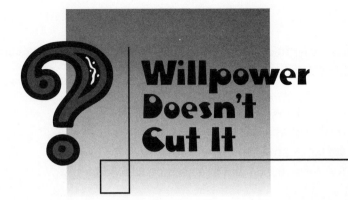

Willpower Doesn't Cut It

Trying to make yourself do the things you want to do by using sheer willpower or mental force, is never a long-term solution to anything. Willpower comes from the logical side of your brain. Remember, that's the side which controls learned and forced action based on times when you are fully aware and in control of your thinking (meaning your conscious thought). This sounds great but, unfortunately, most of our actions are automatic and not consciously thought out.

If you eat food when you're upset just to make yourself feel better, then you need to create good, healthy and automatic responses to the emotional challenges that may currently draw you to food for comfort. Keep in mind, you can't take away an emotional response file without replacing it with another one... And, hopefully, a better one. Your new activity to replace eating food in times of distress could be anything from taking a walk, playing sports of some kind, reading, listening to music, going for a drive, or focusing on a new project or hobby. As long as you don't use food to make yourself feel better, any action is a smarter option.

My daughter used to turn to food when she was upset. Now, she walks. She finds she can blow-off a little steam or think through her challenge if she spends a little time alone with herself. Everyone has their own personal emotional outlet. If food has been yours, then we need to face it and change it.

Everything you do in your life is connected in some way. It is what the theory of "cause and effect" works upon. Every one of your actions during the day affects another. Then, that action will affect still another. Usually these "cause and effect" actions work in a circle and eventually return to affect the initial action. Here is an example:

> You eat poorly, you don't feel well.
> You don't feel well, you are not as productive.
> You are not as productive, you feel stressed.
> You feel stressed, you turn to inappropriate food for comfort.

Because all of our actions are related to each other in some way, we cannot make changes through sheer willpower. Willpower will only help you temporarily and usually for one time only. The next time you face the same kind of challenge, your regular response to that challenge will take over unless you stop to think about it and use your willpower again.

If you want to change your body and maintain the change once you reach your weight goal, then you need to change some of the emotional responses you may have that include using food to boost your happiness level above that emotional median we talked about earlier. Only you know what it takes to make you feel good. Now your new challenge is to find activities to do that are fun and will make you feel better when you find yourself down in the dumps.

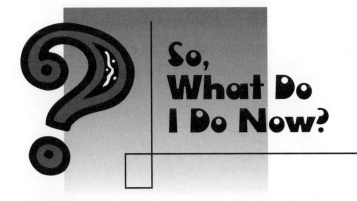

So, What Do I Do Now?

Let's take one step at a time. First, identify your problem. Do you use food for comfort? Do you eat when you're not hungry? Do you eat out of boredom or because you're out with friends? Do you make smart food choices or are you into fast food?

Next, write down every possible thing in your life that may contribute to your weight problem. Even if you think it's dumb or not that big a deal, write it down. Read each item on your list and take one challenge at a time. Now, decide what you see as your goal and think of solutions to the problems that apply to you. While you are finding acceptable solutions that you feel you can live with, think about how you are going to feel once your problem is solved. I bet that thought put a smile on your face already!

Throughout this book I will give you the tools you can use to plan what you need to do and what changes you need to make in order for you to reach your goal. Obviously, you cannot continue to live your life the way you are currently living it, eating the way you are currently eating, and expect to magically lose weight. You have to make the changes...YOU make it happen.

chapter two

Yes You Can and You Will

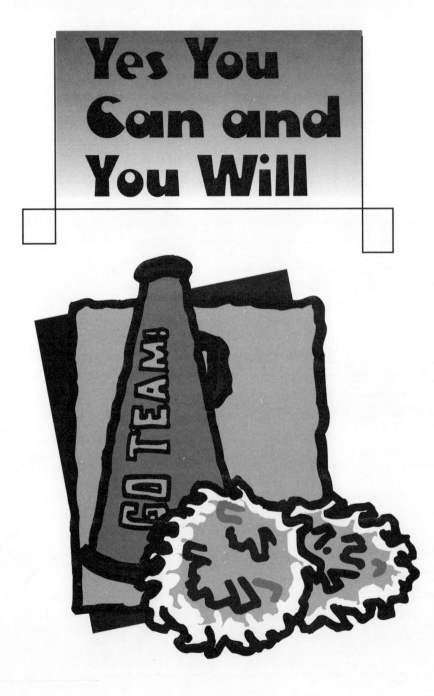

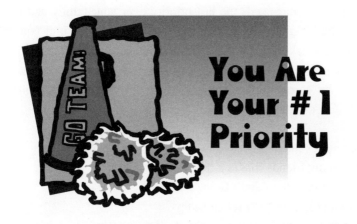

You Are Your # 1 Priority

In a world of hectic schedules, obligations with friends and school, we can sometimes forget about ourselves. Keep in mind, you are your biggest asset AND your biggest responsibility. I think you have learned through this book so far, that being healthy is not just a physical condition. The mind plays a far more important role in our overall health than any other factor. We know, all too well, that we can make ourselves physically ill by allowing ourselves to be over-stressed, confused or mentally exhausted. Now all we need to work on is learning to tell ourselves to be optimistic so that we can start to feel great!

The littlest thing may spoil what could be a great day. Think about this example: You can have two identical days of school. Same classes, same basic assignments, same decent grades, and same schedule. If a friend makes a comment on day two that upsets you in some way, then day one was a "good day" and day two was a "bad day." Even though 99% of both days were identical, your mind decided that one bad word had the ability to ruin your whole day. See how important your mind's evaluation and perception is now?

Don't make your needs the last priority over your family and friends. Likewise, don't start believing that the world revolves around you either. Life is give and take. If you feel that people are taking advantage of you, do something about it. It is amazing how much stress and resentment can be eliminated by correcting uncomfortable or unacceptable situations. Ask yourself a few questions like:

What makes me happy?
Why do my friends frustrate me?
Why do I feel like I don't fit in?
How can I improve my relationships?
What do I want?

Then make a few changes to create balance in your life.

Since so many parts of your life are connected with others around you, be sure to appreciate their assistance. You may need someone to drive you to a friend's house, or to take you to get a new outfit for an upcoming dance. All of the things that are important to you, may not be as important to someone else whose help you need in order to get your own priorities met, so think about others, too.

Taking care of YOU is not a selfish act. When you neglect yourself, you are not the complete person you need and want to be. Your body and what you put into it is one of the main things you can control. Recognizing that you are not happy with how you look and feel is half the battle. Having enough love and appreciation for yourself to do something about it is very admirable. It takes courage to make changes. Courage does not always come naturally to us. That's why more than 50% of Americans are over-weight and getting six percent larger every year!

In order to learn to care for yourself, you need to think about all the different parts that come together to make up your life and evaluate what the good parts and bad parts are. Good nutrition, exercise, stress management, relaxation, visualization and even recognizing that you're making progress toward your goals, all play an important role in your overall happiness and physical condition. Once again, it is all about balance. Your day cannot be constantly made up of all work, or all family, or all play, or all after school activities. You need an ongoing blend of all these things to be a well-rounded person. That is what gives you balance in life.

Live each day in the "now." That means don't sacrifice the fun you know you can have today for the fun you think you might have tomorrow. What if tomorrow's promise doesn't come? When you create the right balance for each day, you will end the day with a feeling of satisfaction and completion. This fact is also true of your weight loss efforts.

Celebrate each pound that you lose rather than constantly thinking about hitting your final weight goal. When I had 85 pounds to lose, 1 would get discouraged if I only lost a pound or two. To finally be 85 pounds lighter seemed light-years away! But, once I realized that every pound that I lost was a success story all by itself, and by acknowledging I was a pound lighter today than yesterday, it gave me the motivation I needed to move forward and keep trying. I knew, no matter what the final outcome was, right NOW I was doing great and I had no reason to think that I would not continue to do great each and every day.

Learn to think positively. Find the good in all things around you. When you cannot see the 'good' in a situation, then either change it or find a positive angle to it that you can consider. Negative energy breeds negative energy so learn to exorcise negativity from your life.

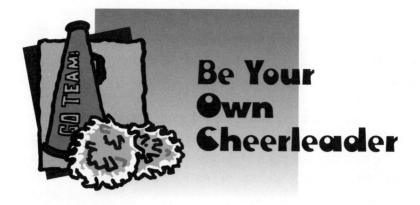

Be Your Own Cheerleader

It's hard to stay motivated when you want to reach your goal so badly and it seems that it may take longer than you'd like. When you share your plans with family and friends, they can help encourage you. Don't keep your weight loss efforts a secret just in case you don't succeed. When you believe you can succeed, you will! Share your faith in your success with everyone you know and let them support you, too. Be sure everyone knows what you expect from them, and exactly how they can help you. You are now in the game of "Lose Weight NOW!" Like any good game, you need an objective, goal, rules for direction and support. If the best thing your family can do for you is to BACK OFF! and let you find your own way, no problem. Just tell them that so they don't frustrate you further.

You need to plan your weight control activities with YOU in mind, not anyone else. Learn to be responsible for yourself and the achievement of your dreams. If a well-meaning friend dumps water on the picture you have created in your mind to be a size 6, try to be understanding and say nothing. A heckler often has their own ax to grind and may be jealous of your success. Your friend may have his or her own agenda and not want you to improve yourself.

Here are a few tips on becoming your own best motivator:

Remove the obstacles obstructing each goal. You can do anything you want to do if you make up your mind to do it. If you want to walk each day, but don't like to walk at night, start early in the morning or after school. You can make it work if you really want to.

Set goals that feel right and work toward them. Don't try to make unrealistic goals for yourself. Know what you're trying to accomplish and how you intend to accomplish it. Plans work much better than wishes. With a plan, you control the outcome.

Admit past failures and find workable solutions. When you control your hunger and elevate your metabolism by eating in a healthy and balanced manner, weight loss can be fast and easy. Don't beat yourself up mentally because you have not been successful losing weight in the past. Now you have the tools you need and you're doing everything right. This time you will succeed!

Think positive thoughts. Negative thoughts can have the same visualization power as positive ones, only in reverse. When you think negative thoughts about yourself such as, "I have no willpower," it can become a self-fulfilling prophecy. Don't let this happen to you. Remove all negative thoughts or limiting beliefs you may have about yourself. Look at the good in everything you do. Don't be angry at yourself for splurging a little. Recognize that you are eating less of most of your problem foods than you have in the past, and it's okay to have a special treat now and then.

I also want you to keep in mind that people will treat you the way you ask to be treated. If you're like most kids, you have probably been pretty lame about telling people what's important to you. For some reason, I bet you think that you're being selfish when you talk about your own needs. But, guess what? You're not being selfish at all. This is your time to shine. You have a vision, a plan and a goal for yourself. That step alone is something to be proud of. You have made a commitment to making changes for the better in your life and people should know about it. Don't let anyone stand in your way of achieving your goals. You have the power inside you right now to do anything that you believe that you can do...USE IT!

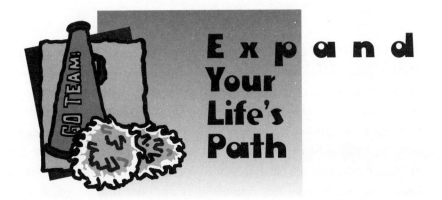

Expand Your Life's Path

Most people are afraid of things that are unknown which usually makes them follow a narrow path in life. As a teenager, everything in your world is pretty well defined for you by your parents. You may move forward each day without a thought about the broad width of life's options, because the unknown is unfamiliar and scary or, you just may not know what questions to ask to find out what else is out there waiting for you.

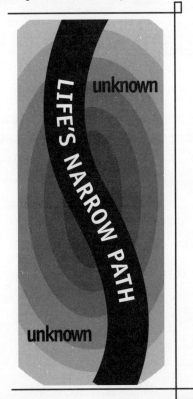

People who live in fear of too many choices may tell themselves that the narrow path (or limiting path) in life is better so they don't have to face options that would make them question or re-evaluate their current belief systems. As an example, some people stay in unpleasant jobs because they know exactly what to expect, even if their job doesn't make them happy. They're afraid that if they got another job, they won't know for certain that things will be better, so they stay where they are. Since there is no absolute guarantee that a job change will make them happier, they decide to stay on the narrow path, knowing that it is an unrewarding and unpleasant job experience.

This same kind of example may apply to you in one form or another. Maybe, your current circle of friends is not the most supportive group of people in the world or they may not have the best health habits either. If you honestly think about it, maybe associating with a group (like the one you may be with now) might have helped you create some of your negative and limiting beliefs. Or, some of the bad eating habits you're trying to break came from the behaviors of the group you want to fit in with. I know you are thinking that because they are your friends, you have a sense of loyalty to them and don't want to criticize. That is a great way for you to be. But, try and look at your friends from the outside and don't be defensive about who they are. Are these people the best influence you could have when you're trying to help better yourself or are their friendships somewhat destructive to you?

This is where the narrow path comes in. Since you know what to expect from your current friends, even if your expectation is pretty low, it still keeps you safely on your narrow and familiar path. Be aware that the path you're on can become a false comfort zone if you stay on it blindly. Take a chance and expand your circle of friends to include some of the people that may be in the 'unknown' sections of your life's path. If your friends are really friends, they won't be upset with your desire to have a wider assortment of friends. Maybe they'll even join you in expanding their relationships, too!

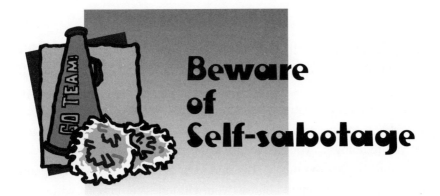

Beware
of
Self-sabotage

I'm sure you are already aware that some people hide behind their weight. Being overweight causes all kinds of emotional triggers and can also help a lot of people to justify their incorrect beliefs about themselves that interfere with their weight loss efforts. I want you to really understand how damaging this can be if you have this kind of fear because fear may be part of another emotional file that will cause you to sabotage all the great efforts you are making in order to have positive changes in your life.

Here's the deal: When the logical side of your brain communicates with the emotional side, it creates what professionals call "an inner dialogue." It's like you're talking to yourself about yourself in your head. If you do not control your inner dialogue by using healthy and positive beliefs that you have collected in your files along the way, your inner dialogue can project negative thoughts. Any doubt you may have about your ability to achieve weight loss success can cause negative thoughts to be directed toward your current weight loss efforts. This is especially true if you have unsuccessfully tried to reach your weight goal in the past. Remember, since your brain only believes what you tell it to believe, you can successfully lose weight if YOU think you can really do it.

Our inner dialogue communicates with us when we are in our weakest condition. It may tell us we are incapable of success and remind us that we have failed at so many other programs before, that we may start to believe that it is a real possibility that this will only be another failed attempt to shed our extra pounds.

If you're not careful, your inner dialogue can be very mean and always remind you of all the limitations you may think you have. If it's not stopped by you changing your thinking, constantly telling yourself that you may not be successful will cause you to begin to support that belief. Hidden somewhere in an emotional file may already be your feeling that you are incapable of weight loss success. Without even realizing that you're doing it, you may begin to act in a way that guarantees your failure, like eating too much. Because your actions will always support your beliefs, if your mind believes you will fail, your actions will make sure that you do.

Knowing you can control your thoughts will really help you to think in a "can do" manner. When you begin to only let your brain accept positive thought patterns, your inner dialogue will become positive and support your efforts, rather than negative and destructive. If you begin to remove all limiting beliefs that say "I can't, I can't" from your life, then your inner dialogue will have no more negative files left on the emotional side of your brain that it can pull from. Once the files are gone, there is nothing available to sabotage your goals.

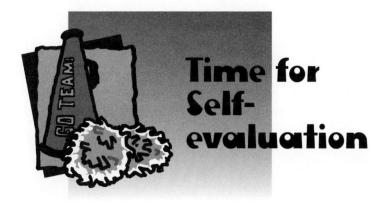

Time for Self-evaluation

Since all the different parts of your life are connected to each other in some way, you must figure out what conditions or eating habits have caused you to be overweight in the first place. Once you know what you think is the source of your weight problem, then we can deal directly with all the things you may need to do in order to make permanent changes. As long as you live and eat the same way while you are losing weight as you plan to live and eat after the weight is gone (and it will be gone soon!), then you will have no reason to ever gain the weight back again.

Be honest about what you believe has caused you to be unhappy with how you look and feel. Face those beliefs and either change them or find solutions so they don't continue to screw up your plans for yourself. Change is sometimes frightening but it is worth it. It is about getting more mature, improving who you are and growing as a person. Change is about taking another look at the walls you've built around yourself and expanding your world. You can change anything within your control that you decide you need to change. That includes your bad habits, too. When you find better options for habits that you know are not right or healthy for you, make those new options the ones you like the most. It's just as easy to make eating healthy foods become your favorite as it is to continue to make excuses for eating food that is not very good for you. You control your choices, so you control your habits. And, remember, making the right choice always gives you a sense of pride and accomplishment as an added bonus.

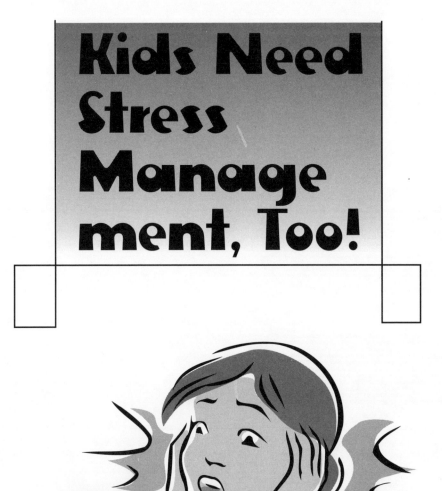

chapter three

Kids Need Stress Management, Too!

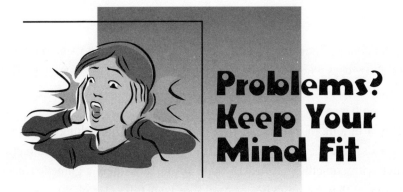

Problems?
Keep Your
Mind Fit

Even though kids and young adults know better, they often associate stress with their parents' world. But even experts recognize that more and more kids are "stressed out" and have a hard time keeping up with all the pressures and craziness of every day life. Sound familiar?

Stress can come in all forms. School is certainly very demanding. Even if learning comes easy for you, there are still pressures being thrown at you from all sides. Add feeling a little insecure about your appearance or body size and the stress level meter moves up a lot!

I've worked with kids who try to juggle a full academic load while participating in an extra-curricular activity just about every day of the week. One day is swim practice, another day soccer, choir, drama, or band practice. Between extra-curricular activities, enrichment programs and after-school lessons coupled with chores at home and homework assignments, who wouldn't feel overwhelmed and run ragged (I know your mother does!). And you haven't even made time yet for a social life...no pressure there!

You may even feel you have "over-achiever" type parents that seem to be pushing you into a fast-paced lifestyle that is really more suited for them than it is for you. But, what do you expect? All parents want their children to be more successful than they are - it's human nature. Don't get mad, communicate. Don't let their expectations frustrate you to the point of depression, headaches, eating disorders, inability to focus or just a general lack of enthusiasm or disinterest in life.

You have a mouth. Instead of filling it full of food to get back at your parents for wanting the best for you, COMMUNICATE. I know, easier said than done. "They don't listen," is a common complaint from today's teens. But, guess what? You may not think your parents are listening. In fact, they may appear to be arguing and disagreeing when, in reality, they actually do hear you.

Hey, I'm a mom. There are times I'd rather die than admit that one of my kids gave me a very rational argument that was clearly in direct conflict with something I wanted them to do...and their argument was more logical than my thinking. And, like your folks, I probably yelled and ranted and raved to make my points without taking the time to consider theirs. But, after walking away, I really began to think about what my son or daughter had to say and I am always influenced by them. When they rationally communicate with me on a regular basis, it creates a pattern to promote my listening rather than my reacting.

Communication needs to come from both sides, too. It's not easy growing up and it's not easy BEING grown up. You are responsible for your life but, as parents, we feel responsible for your life. It's not always easy for your parents to let go enough to let you find your own way.

But, in order for your parents to allow you extra freedom to show that you are responsible enough to make some of your own decisions, you need to show them that you are able to assume that responsibility. Your actions need to demonstrate your ability to show responsible thinking so that your parents can trust your judgement. Life is no different than having a job. When you hit the job market, you are only going to be hired for a position that your boss feels you are able to do. Likewise, your parents are not going to trust your judgement if you never show them that you have any.

Getting your body 'together' requires that you get all-of-you 'together.' That means you start with your head and work your way down. Attitude is everything. If you feel stuck in a circle of negativity and are not sure how to get out, you're not alone. Every day, millions of Americans feel depressed or suffer from some type of energy "zapper" that drains the life out of them. Sometimes it's hard to get out of the circle because your negative thoughts can leave you without motivation or enough energy to make the improvements you may need to make in order to get back on track. Well, it's possible to reverse the cycle...NOW!

While negative thoughts can lead to negative actions, the opposite is also true. A positive outlook can lead to positive actions. If you find that you just can't get your head in the right place to start, you can try taking action first, then your mood is sure to follow.

When life hands you a basket of lemons, learn to make lemonade! Certain ways of acting can lead to positive mental health and a happier outlook. Practicing "happy thinking" can help you keep a positive attitude and deal with stress.

Here are a few positive actions you can try to get you jump-started right away:

1. **Accept and care for yourself.** No one is perfect, not even gorgeous models and movie stars. You are a unique indvid ual so focus on the positive parts of your personality and accept who you are. What do you like about yourself? What do your friends like about you? Are you dependable and loyal to the peo ple you care about? Isn't being counted on by the people you care about the most important trait   you can have?

2. **Take responsibility for your life.**   I'm not suggesting you necessarily start paying rent, but, control what is in your power to control. You are responsible for your actions, nobody else is. Start making decisions about who you are and who you want to be. Pattern your daily activities around becoming the person your vision says you can become.

3. **Accept that life is a mixture of good and bad.** Everyone has ups and downs. Accept that things don't always happen as you'd like them to. Life can sometimes be unfair. Maybe   one of your disappointments is directly related to something your parents could not avoid. Try to see other sides of situations instead of personalizing everything and assuming   nobody care enough to consider your needs.

4. **Be flexible.** This is probably the most important thing you can learn in life. Flexibility isn't just needed for the years that you're living at home. You will need to be flexible forever. Learn to change what you can and adjust to what you can't change. If you don't learn to bend, you'll break.

5. **Enjoy the moment.** Life is made up of moments. Some good, some bad. Some happy, some sad. If you take time to enjoy and embrace the good and happy moments, they will become the treasure chest of memories for you to draw upon later in life.

6. **Express your feelings.** Always be open about your emotions, both positive and negative. Communicate. Don't be afraid. You may not get the response you are initially expecting. If you have not been much of a communicator in the past, you're going to have to teach the people you are with that you have a desire to make a communication change. Expressing your feelings in a constructive and positive manner is part of being human. If someone can't handle your honesty, then something is wrong with them and not you. If you have a hard time talking about your feel ings, then write them down instead. Writing allows you to say exactly how you feel and forces the reader to "hear" exactly what you're trying to say. They can't interrupt. They can't argue (yet). At least, through writing, you have the chance to say how you feel without fearing what the other person will do while you're speaking. The conflict about whatever is bothering you may still ultimately arise between the two of you, but at least you know you have made your feelings on the subject very clear. And, sometimes, writing down your feelings makes you take another look at them to see if they were as important as you really thought. When you're open-minded, even with yourself, your own position on the matter-at-hand may change too.

7. **Balance your life.** Don't run over yourself trying to cram too much into each day. Learn to balance family, friends, school, homework and outside activities. Take time to rest and think about the good things that are happening to you. If any one activity begins to take on too much importance or takes up too much of your time, re-evaluate its contribution to your life and the direction you're beginning to map out for yourself. The tele phone, for example, may not be the priority when you have homework still pending! (Wow! Do I sound like a mom, what???)

8. **Develop interests that stimulate you.** Find positive outlets for your energy instead of using food to pass away the time. Experiment with healthy options until you find something you enjoy.

9. **Think creatively.** Work out solutions to your problems. Don't just accept what happens to you and get depressed or frustrated. When a big problem arises, take a deep breath and move forward. Figure out what other options you may have. Be open-minded and not judgmental. Honestly look at all sides of the situation and have a complete understanding of how this problem could have been created or avoided in order to eliminate the chance of it happening again.

10. **Work toward your goal.** Recognize your accomplishments. See every little positive action as a success. Every pound you lose is a success. Don't always dwell on the end result. Sometimes the final goal seems too far away to stay motivated day-to-day. When you recognize and acknowledge your own achievements, big or small, you will soon see how easy it can be to overcome just about any potential obstacle....just take each day one day at a time!

The one thing you can control in this crazy world is yourself, so start with basic organization. Have a plan for your day that includes smart eating. For what it's worth, a balanced diet can eliminate being tired or the inability to think. Junk food is neither brain-food nor good for you, so find the time to eat smart and healthy foods. How can you expect to be productive when you're tired and have a hard time paying attention?

If you have not been much of a healthy eater up until now, you're not alone. According to one of the pediatric journals, only 1% of young people aged 2-19 have healthy diets! It also reported that the same group of kids tested on average, received 40% of their energy from fat and sugar items like candy bars or chips.

Stress management is a fancy term for time management, too. The two go together like shoes & socks. Make time to finish your homework and complete your assigned responsibilities. You know you're going to have to do them anyway, so why make more trouble and stress for yourself? Don't take advantage of curfew times and make your parents worry or get upset with you unnecessarily. Take time to talk to them about things that concern you BEFORE those concerns become real issues. Nobody likes surprises.

And, for heaven's sake, don't take on more activities than you can handle. Not only does trying to cram too much into your daily calendar add a lot of additional frustration and pressure on yourself, trying to juggle the time management factors that go with all these activities usually means that regular meals go right out the window. It's fast-food time because you only have a few minutes between planned activities to snarf down something that will keep you going and energized through the rest of your day.

Staying in control isn't just about what you eat. It's also about controlling your life. Raise your standards. Learn to like living, feeling and looking better. Hold on to your vision and always keep it close to you. With just a little planning to make that vision into reality, all the other pieces will fall right into place.

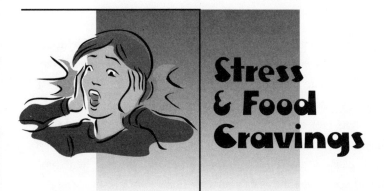

Stress & Food Cravings

I'm sure by now, you're probably more than aware that stress is certainly a condition that triggers food cravings. But, it is also important for you to be aware that your cravings may also be caused by some necessary vitamin, mineral or nutrient that may be missing in your body. When your body has something missing, (a deficiency), it craves the kinds of food that contains whatever it needs to replace what is missing - even if it's sugar.

A lot has been written by doctors on food cravings, but nothing is known for sure about these "irresistible urges" that some people get for certain foods. Chocolate and other foods are not addictive in the same way that alcohol or cigarettes are, but anytime somebody feels they "need" to eat these foods (and that's just about all they can think about until they do) it almost feels like an addiction. Painful, physical withdrawal symptoms do not result if you cut out a food entirely. But, like true addictions, food cravings can be damaging, especially for people trying to lose weight or control diabetes.

Many professionals believe that cravings have a biological basis, which is a fancy way of saying your body is telling your brain that it needs to eat something in particular. Out-of-control hormones, such as insulin in the case of diabetics cause cravings. Let me give you an example. I'm sure if you're female, you may have had food cravings, probably for sugary stuff, just around the time of your menstrual period because your hormones are raging. But, at least from a medical standpoint, no research on the subject has found any clear-cut association between food cravings and hormone levels.

Another theory is that food cravers are trying to correct some chemical imbalance they may have in their body. Eating pickles or potato chips, for instance, can make up for a sodium deficiency. Experts say that depressed people will overdose on sweets because eating a lot of gooey carbohydrates promotes the release of serotonin, a "feel good" brain chemical, which gives them an almost immediate sense of happiness and well being. DON'T GET ANY NEW IDEAS ABOUT THAT...JUST KEEP READING!

The best defense for a food craving is common sense. First and foremost, recognize the craving for what it is then deal with it. Don't pretend it will go away, because it won't. You know, first hand, that the items you know you should not eat are the ones you want first.

Be smart. Have low-fat, low-calorie replacements for the kind of foods you crave readily available. Nobody thinks a 30-calorie fudge pop is going to replace a big bowl of Häagen-Dazs ice cream...but it is certainly better than not having ice cream at all. Even if you eat the entire box of fudge pops, you will be eating less fat and less calories than eating the pint of ice cream.

You can handle any food challenge if you face it heads-up and are prepared. Don't have the items you don't want to eat sitting in your refrigerator, or nearby. It's a lot easier to make the right food choices when you limit your options to only good stuff!

Be sure that before you eat something you don't think you should, that you think about the reason you're going to eat it. Is eating a big donut your choice because you want it, or are you eating it as a reaction to something else going on in your life that you'd rather not face? You have control! Your brain is programmed like the memory on a computer with all your beliefs based on your lessons and your experiences. You can certainly figure out what's really drawing you to the refrigerator and snack shop.

As you learn more about yourself and what makes you act the way you do, your belief system will change. In a very short time, many of your old 'files' will be reworked or discarded. Change is good. Reading this book is about change. Your interest has been peaked and you're already well on your way to recognizing that you can accomplish anything you set your mind to so don't let stress overwhelm you. Take control. Something you need to deal with is just something you need to deal with whether it's a "good something" or a "bad something." So, just try to deal with it by using as little emotion as possible. Extra upset will only get in your way.

chapter four

Think Yourself Thin

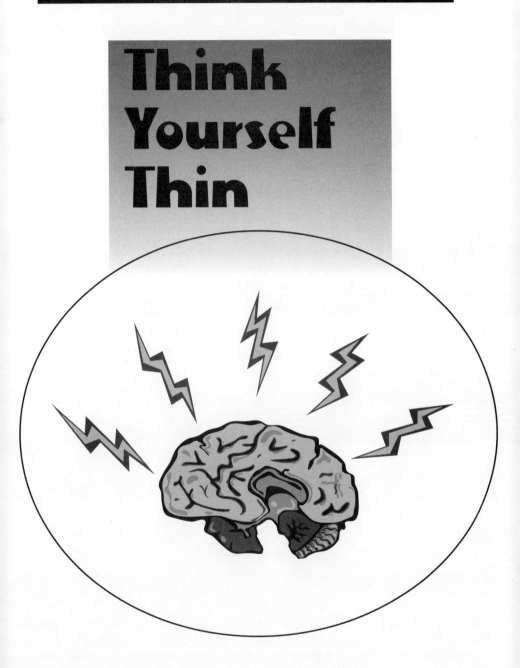

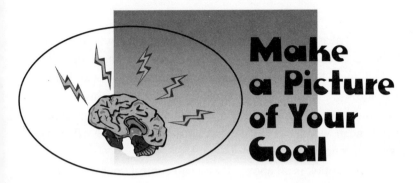

Make a Picture of Your Goal

Now that you know more about how your brain works and you are learning that you can create any reality or result you believe you can create, what you now need to do is create a picture in your mind of how you would like to look and feel in a new body. Pictures or visualizations are very powerful mind exercises. They send signals to the brain that come from your imagination or memories. When you create this picture in your mind, you will start to build more emotional files that are tied to the picture. You will experience, through your imagination, how you will feel when you are thinner and how people will react to your new appearance. You will also learn to feel confident and self-assured.

When you think about the picture or image you want to create, the brain actually reconstructs or builds the pattern of nerve cell activity that takes place every time you put this picture in your memory. By thinking about your picture over and over for about a month, all the feelings that you put with your picture will then go into your emotional filing cabinets to tell your body how to respond.

Let me give you an example of how your mind can make your body react. When you dream, your dreams draw pictures from your memory and that is why they appear so real to you. When you're dreaming, your brain can't tell the difference between something that is really happening and something that is only your imagination. When you dream you are being chased, your heart beats faster and harder just like it would if you were really being chased. Even your arms and legs may show signs of running or kicking. Because your brain really thought it was being chased when you were dreaming, your body thought it was being chased even though you never left your bed and were sound asleep at the time. That is what I mean when I say that what you think can and will ultimately control your body.

This is what this book is all about. If you can control your mind, you can control your mouth! If you allow yourself to see how great you really are and let yourself acknowledge how much greater you can be if you want to, then you can see that you are the master of your own destiny! I am the first person to tell you that just thinking about a change of appearance will not make that change happen. But, thinking about the change, picturing the change and making a plan to make the picture become your new reality is very achievable.

If you have a picture in your mind of what you want to look like, all you need to do is live like your picture is already real. That means if you want to look different, you need to eat differently. You need to eat like the person in your picture would eat. Maybe you need to exercise or even act differently. You can't continue to eat like a heavy person and expect to become a thin one. But, if you figure out the changes that you need to make in your life that are getting in the way of making your picture real, and then make a commitment to make those changes. You will be surprised at how quickly your body responds.

See it...Believe it...Make it happen.

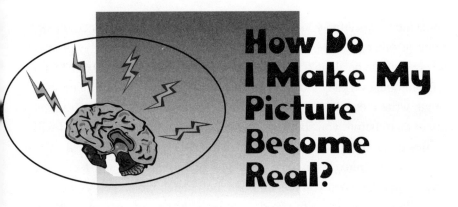

How Do I Make My Picture Become Real?

OK, time to make a picture of a "new you" in your head. If you have been overweight for most of your young life and you are having a difficult time imagining yourself looking differently than you do now, then find a picture of someone in a magazine that looks like you want to look. Be realistic in your choice. If you are 5' tall, don't select the body of a 6' model to be your picture. You must believe that the picture you are creating for yourself is one that you can actually work to make real. If you start off with an unrealistic expectation and you know in your heart that you're never going to look like the picture you've made of yourself in your mind, then your efforts are doomed before you begin.

Each time you do the exercise, your mind needs to take you through the same memory patterns. The reason you want to think the same things in the same way every day is simple: I want you to constantly recreate your picture in your mind until it becomes a strong memory in your brain. Your brain will then begin to actually experience what you are telling it you see, and start making all the positive emotional files you will need to support your picture with actions. When the picture becomes real to your brain, it becomes real to your body just like in my dream example.

Creating the picture of your new image is very personal. It needs to be done at a time when you won't have any interruptions or chores that someone is expecting you to take care of. Turn off your pager, cell phone, radio or other possible disturbance. Go into your room, a park, or anywhere you can be alone with yourself. Be comfortable and relaxed. Don't let common, everyday thoughts get in your way. If you have a lot on your mind, write those thoughts down on a piece of paper so you won't forget about them before you start this exercise. By doing that, your mind will be free of anything that may get in the way of focusing on your goal. You only want to think about how your new body will look and feel...how great it will be when you are slimmer...how much more energy you will have...how eating unhealthy foods will get in the way of your goal. While you are thinking about all of these things, your brain will be creating all the positive files that you will associate with your new self.

Keep focusing your mind on these very specific, empowering thoughts. Disregard everyday, conscious interruptions and just let yourself experience the thought. Let your imagination touch it, smell it, see it, hear it. Experience how strong and empowered you feel when you imagine your picture becoming a reality.

You need to do this exercise each day for a month and for about thirty minutes each time. When your thoughts focus on creating a new body, you will imagine yourself shrinking. You will begin to sense how you will feel when you are thinner. You will experience how other people will react to your being thinner and looking fit.

When you are using meditation-type music to help you clear your mind, and you find that you become so relaxed during this exercise that you fall asleep, don't worry. The work can still be done if you're sleeping as well as when you are awake.

Living your picture becomes the final step. Everyone needs to identify what needs to happen and what steps need to be taken in order for their picture of themselves to become a reality. When your goal is to lose weight, you will plan what lifestyle changes, if any, you'll need to make. How will you need to change what you eat or maybe even when you eat it? Is exercise going to be needed for you to achieve your new image? The answers to all of these questions will be covered in this book, so if you're up to it...turn the page!

chapter five

Plan Your Changes

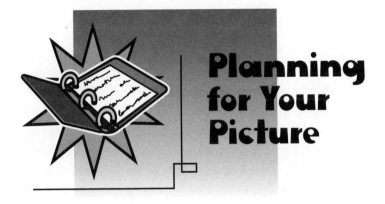

Planning for Your Picture

This is the fun part. This is where you will take a good hard look at what you are doing now that keeps you from losing unwanted pounds and inches, what you should be doing, and what changes you need to make in order to have the body you want. Be very honest. You can't fool yourself.

This part of the book is designed to help you create a picture of your new image, then plan what steps you'll need to take to break the patterns that have kept you away from being the person in your picture up until now. You always have options. Once you start to put your plan into action, feel comfortable that your plans can change. Your personal commitment to making all of this work and how you follow your plan is up to you.

Fill out Part 1 and 2 of the questionnaire in this book before you begin to create your picture. Since it is very important that you believe that your goal is attainable, beginning to plan for it will help you to become a real believer. Making it happen is not that tough when you see it written down in black and white. It will also help you be certain of your goal. Once you are comfortable that your "picture-of-a-thinner-you" is set firmly in place, complete the remaining parts of the worksheets.

Keep in mind that this same exercise can be used for any goal you have. No matter what the goal, it is important that your answers are specific. In other words, if the question asks "What health improvements would you like to see? Do you want to be more active, have more energy, feel better?" Don't answer that question with a simple "Have more energy" answer. Be specific. Write down exactly HOW you want to have more energy. Your answer should read something like, "Have enough energy to exercise when I get home from school, not need a nap in the afternoon, and stay awake at night to enjoy TV with my family." With a complete answer, you'll really know what you're trying to accomplish.

Writing down your plans works a whole lot better than just thinking about them. A written plan gives you something you can look at, think about and change when it's not working the way you want it to. It also becomes a type of diary so you can start to chart your success because you WILL be successful!

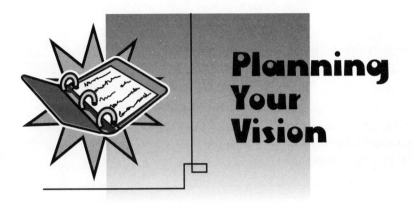

Planning Your Vision

1. KNOW YOUR OUTCOME AND SET YOUR VISION

Now that you have identified your goals and believe that they are achievable, take a moment to think about and list why these goals are important to you. You also want to be clear about what you think may have happened that got you to your current weight so you can avoid duplicating those same actions or conditions in the future.

a. What is your ultimate weight loss goal?

_____
_____
_____
_____

b. What would you like to accomplish in the next 3 months?

_____
_____
_____
_____
_____

c. What would you like to accomplish in the next 6-12 months?

_____

_____

_____

_____

d. What health improvements would you like to see? Do you want to be more active, have more energy, feel better?

_____

_____

_____

_____

_____

_____

e. How will you feel when you achieve your goal? Will looking better make you feel more confident? Happier? Proud of yourself for getting the job done?

_____

_____

_____

_____

_____

f. How will others look at you when you are thinner? Will your family be proud? Your friends? Potential dates?

_____

_____

_____

_____

_____

_____

g. How would you change the way you'll live once you reach your goal weight? Will you need to exercise more? Eat out less? Have less fast-food?

_____

_____

_____

_____

_____

_____

_____

_____

2. KNOW YOUR REASONS WHY

Understanding what the deal is about any challenge that comes your way is the key to solving it. If you don't figure out the cause of your problems, how can you expect to fix them? By being clear about your history and the bad habits you may have developed in the past, you have taken a giant step toward making sure that you will not self-sabotage your current self-improvement efforts.

a. Why do you think you are overweight?

_____

_____

_____

- -

b. Why is achieving your goal important to you?

_____

_____

_____

- -

c. Why are you concerned about your current physical condition?

_____

_____

_____

d. Why is it important to you how other people see you?

_____

_____

- -

3. TAKE ACTION - Make It Happen!

This is the challenging part: Planning what you are willing to do to make your picture come true. Don't make this part overwhelming. List your overall plans but only make small changes each week until you feel you are able to do more. The more realistic you are about making the changes you need to make, a little bit at a time, the easier all the changes will be for you to handle.

a. What has to happen in order for you to achieve your goal? What changes in your snacking or dealing with stress do you need to make? Must you eliminate some of the junk foods? Stop ordering "biggie" sized portions? Eat more fruit? Eat more balanced meals?

_____

_____

_____

_____

_____

b. What will your biggest eating challenges be that you will need to overcome? Snacking? Binging? Late-night eating?

_____

_____

_____

_____

c. What lifestyle changes do you need to make? Less fast-food? Exercise?

_____

_____

_____

_____

_____

d. What are you going to do this week to help you toward your goal? Go to the gym? Take your lunch to school? Find better snack options?

_____

_____

_____

_____

_____

e. What activity are you going to do just for YOU this week?

_____

_____

_____

_____

_____

4. EVALUATE YOUR SUCCESS

This is the most important part of your process: Checking out how you're doing. Every pound, every inch, every bad eating habit that you change that benefits your body, all add up to bring balance and happiness back into your life. Do not take these changes lightly, no matter how small they may seem. Every change shows your dedication to a "New You." Watch it happen. Now you can see for yourself what a powerful and successful person you really can be because the changes in your body are there for all the world to see, too.

a. How much smaller are you getting?

_____

_____

_____

_____

b. What food changes have you made that you won't miss or go back to later?

_____

_____

_____

_____

c. How much 'junk food' have you cut from your diet? Do you eat smaller helpings and not large portions anymore?

_____

_____

_____

_____

d. How do you feel physically?

_____

_____

_____

_____

e. Do you feel you have more energy now?

_____

_____

_____

f. Are you exercising pretty often?

_____

_____

_____

g. Are people beginning to notice a difference in your appearance?

_____

_____

_____

h. Are you happy with your progress?

_____

_____

_____

i. What do you need to do now to make your program more successful?

_____

_____

_____

_____

_____

_____

5. ONGOING EVALUATION AND ADJUSTMENT

Be sure you check out your progress weekly and adjust your plan as opportunities pop up along the way. Don't weigh yourself every day. There are a lot of things that affect our daily weight, even outside temperature. You should weigh yourself wearing the same clothes or PJ's one morning each week. You may also want to put a tape measure around your waist to see if you have lost inches when the scales don't seem to be going down.

The eating guide for this program is going to have you focus your meals around proteins like meat, chicken, turkey, and seafood. Sometimes people lose body fat and get leaner but don't see a pound loss. If you feel flabby now, you may have a high body-fat content in relation to your lean muscle mass. By exercising and eating more chicken and meat, you may be shrinking in size but not in weight.

Muscle is five times heavier than fat. When you lose a pound of fat by exercising (which increases muscle), you may find yourself getting smaller in physical size but not in weight. I want you to be aware that this might happen so you're not discouraged when the scale doesn't move as quickly as you would like it to. Looking your best is more important than hitting a target weight number on the scale so don't make the scale your only measure of success. Keep reminding yourself that you're successful every time you eat better food or take better care of your body. Afterall, that's what feeling great is all about.

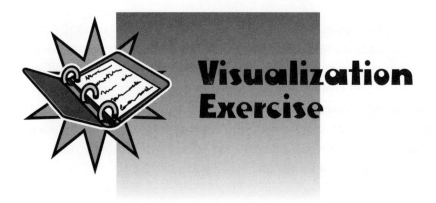

Visualization Exercise

I spoke earlier about finding a picture of yourself when you were thinner, or of someone you would like to look like if you are having a hard time coming up with a mental picture of your thinner self. Sometimes it's a lot easier to create a picture in your mind when you have a picture in your hand to look at first. Keep a copy of your goal picture someplace where you can look at it a lot. Your locker, your bathroom mirror, or by your bed are all good places. Looking at it every day helps keep the picture fresh in your mind. It will also help to motivate you since you know in your heart that you will be looking like the image in your photo one day soon.

Be realistic in your photo selection. Don't use a picture of someone who's body you could never have. If you are a tall, large boned person, do not use a photograph of a tiny or petite person to be your inspiration. Unrealistic pictures will only frustrate and depress you, so don't use them.

You can also place a picture of your own face on top of the magazine picture you cut out. By doing that, you will really "see" yourself as you will look once you reach your goal.

Every time you see a significant difference in your size, take new photographs. Watching yourself shrink and keeping a photo-diary of your progress will also be great motivation.

Place the photo you have found that represents how you would like to look in the box on the left. You can also use an assortment of pictures if you think that will motivate you more. As you begin to actually see and experience your own personal weight loss, place new pictures in the box on the right. It's fun to see your progress and know that you are well on your way to reaching your goal.

PLACE GOAL PHOTO HERE   PLACE AFTER PHOTO HERE

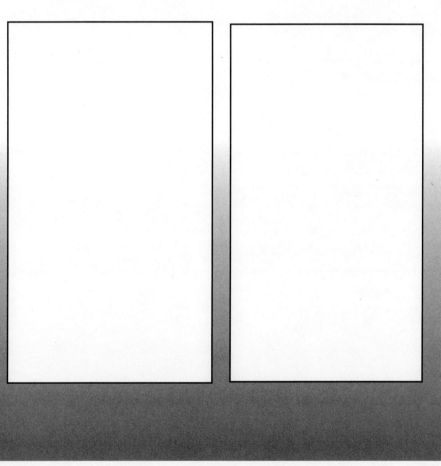

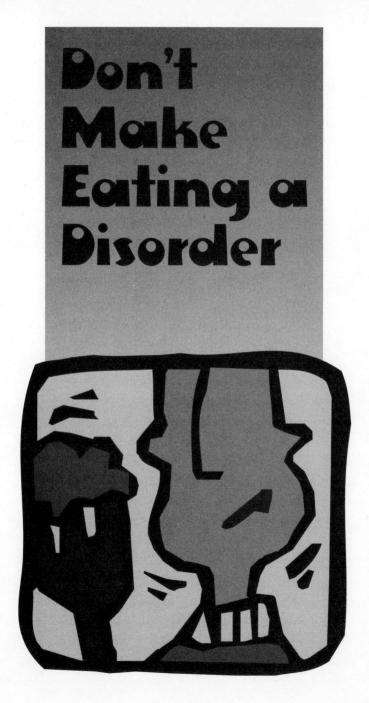

chapter six

Don't Make Eating a Disorder

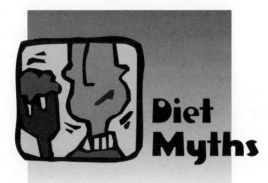

Diet Myths

Now we're going to get down to basics. First, let me assure you that you don't have to be a nutritionist to learn how to eat right. You know more about what you should and shouldn't eat right now than you give yourself credit for.

Starting a weight management program requires two things: A positive attitude and the desire to succeed. If both of these things are in place, you can't help but be successful...no matter what your genetic history of family obesity may be.

Below are some of the most common diet myths that need to be ignored. When you're focused and start to accept the fact that you can accomplish anything you set your mind to, weight loss success will be yours in no time.

Myth #1: IT TAKES TREMENDOUS WILLPOWER TO LOSE WEIGHT. I agree that it isn't always easy to pass up some of the foods that make weight loss difficult, but it doesn't take willpower to find low-calorie or low-fat alternatives for the same item. Since there is no such thing as "off limits food," you can eat anything you want. Just be smart and don't overdo it. If you feel like ice cream, eat frozen yogurt instead. If you want chips, try fat-free pretzels or air popped popcorn. When birthday cake is being passed around, have a small piece instead of the portion that reads "Happy Sweet Sixteenth Birthday Suzanne!" It's not willpower that you need. It's taking credit for the fact that you are learning to make responsible choices about the things you put into your mouth.

Myth #2: IF YOU LOSE WEIGHT, YOU'LL PROBABLY GAIN IT BACK. People only gain their weight back if they were unrealistic about how they lost their weight in the first place. I'm not going to let you go on a liquid diet and lose weight by "drinking your meals" because you're not going to continue to "drink your meals" for the rest of your life. When you want to lose weight permanently, you need to make permanent changes in the way you eat. This may even mean you need to eat more, not less.

You have a system inside your body called your "metabolism." Your metabolism is your body's system to process food and burn calories. Every time you reduce the calories you eat, your metabolic system gets a little slower. If you have dieted your way to a very inactive metabolism, your system is operating so slowly that even eating only 800 calories a day won't help you lose weight.

When you starve yourself and don't eat enough food to keep you healthy, your metabolism shuts down and puts you on a type of self-induced life support. It stores as much fat as it can so vital organs like your heart and liver can continue to function. You need to feed and energize your system regularly so your metabolism can operate as efficiently as possible.

If you think of your body like a sleek sports car (the Jaguar model rather than the "bathtub" Porsche!), just imagine how poorly your car would perform if you failed to give it gas. Well, your body is no different.

When you make lean and healthy food choices that enable your body to lose weight, there is no reason that your new weight cannot be maintained if you keep eating the same way.

Myth # 3: I WAS BORN FAT. I HAVE FAT GENES. You may have fat 'jeans' but nobody is born to be overweight. If obesity runs in your family and it has not been medically explained, then it can probably be explained by the grocery store foods you grew up eating. Overweight parents tend to have overweight children. They teach their children how to be overweight by purchasing and preparing the wrong foods. Even the most dramatic medical condition that causes obesity can usually be overcome if that's what you want to do.

Myth #4: IF YOU REALLY WANT TO LOSE WEIGHT, YOU MUST FOLLOW A STRICT DIET. This is probably the biggest myth of all! Every person will have a different 'diet' they want to follow because every person has a different lifestyle and likes to eat different stuff. What we will accomplish, by the end of this book, is your ability to identify the foods you enjoy the most. We'll find healthy foods you like to eat, problem foods that need to be exchanged on occasion for acceptable alternatives and activities that dictate special foods (like pizza after each football or basketball game) that need to be taken into account, too. Your way of eating while you lose your unwanted pounds and inches will be the same way you're going to eat once you reach your weight loss goal. That's why you aren't going to regain those unwanted pounds!

Myth #5: SINCE IT'S BAD FOR YOU TO GAIN & LOSE & GAIN & LOSE, IT'S SAFER JUST TO STAY HEAVY. Maintaining too much weight for long periods of time is a serious health risk and can even cause premature death. There is no question that gaining and losing weight, over and over, is not healthy. But staying heavy is a much greater risk, not only to your health, but to your self-esteem. It's no fun to be fat or to feel inferior to other people around you. So, DO SOMETHING ABOUT IT!

Myth #6: YOU CAN LOSE WEIGHT JUST BY ELIMINATING FAT FROM YOUR DIET. Keeping fat content low when selecting the food you eat is certainly a great start, but you can't lose weight if you eat more calories than your body is able to burn...whether they are fat calories or not. As a matter of fact, if you eat too much starch like potatoes, rice and pasta which can contain no fat at all, your body can become a fat manufacturing machine. If you don't do enough physical activity during the day to burn up all the sugar that comes from the processing of all that starch, what you don't use turns to fat. Besides, your body needs some fat. "Good fat" not "bad fat." Fat is the body's lubricating oil. If you don't eat some fat, there will be no oils in your body to keep your physical machine going.

"Good fats" are essential fats that are found in nuts, dried beans, meats and the natural oil in fish. If you eat foods like these, you will give your body healthy, natural fats. "Bad fats" are the man-made fats that are found in chips or the shortening used in most commercial cookies, cakes and baked items. It isn't difficult to know what fats to stay away from. When you exercise control in your food selection, most of your "good fat - bad fat" decisions will take care of themselves.

Myth #7: EATING THE SAME LOW CALORIE MENU EVERY DAY WILL HELP ME LOSE WEIGHT FASTER. Nope! Your body likes variety just like your taste buds. Since an elevated metabolism is the key to weight loss, you don't want to do anything to slow it down. Forcing your metabolic system to process the same foods day-in and day-out will slow it down a lot. When you rotate your food and don't eat the same things all the time, it will keep your system much more active and stimulated. Stimulated systems process food better and, eventually, show their efficiency in the form of weight loss, so be creative. If you're having chicken for lunch today, have meat for lunch tomorrow.

Myth #8: IF I JUST GIVE IT TIME, I'LL PROBABLY OUTGROW THIS. It is true that you may be young enough to be fighting additional 'baby fat' but you're not going to outgrow bad habits. You obviously think you have a weight problem right now or you would not be reading this book. If I'm right, it can't hurt to learn a few things that will help you make the most of your fitness potential with food.

Myth #9: WHAT I DRINK HAS NO EFFECT ON MY WEIGHT. Because we think of drinks as liquid that goes right through the body, sometimes we forget that most beverages contain a lot of sugar or calories. Since 1978, kids have doubled their intake of soda and tripled their intake of sweetened fruit drinks. You'd be a lot better off eating the oranges, apples or grapefruits that you intend on juicing rather than drinking them. You'll be a lot fuller and have the value of the vitamins and minerals that are in the pulp of the fruit. It takes about six oranges to make a 5-ounce glass of OJ in the morning. I doubt that you would even consider eating six oranges at one sitting. I strongly recommend saving fruits as something to eat not drink and if you have really made a commitment to losing weight, try drinking good old-fashioned water. Not only does it have remarkable hydrating or water placement properties that provide great benefits to your skin, it's the only liquid that flushes fats from your body! Just think...you can almost drink your way to fitness!

Myth #10: EXERCISE IS THE BEST WAY TO LOSE WEIGHT. It's true that exercise is a great metabolic stimulant and will help your body feel better, perform better and increase fat burn. But the real truth is, you must control the food you put into your body in order for your body to perform in such a way that it allows for weight loss. Exercise is the best answer for toning and strengthening your body and its organs. And, if the right food balance is not provided by you, your body won't recieve the proteins, vitamins and minerals it needs to be healthy and lean. Workouts are great and have their own benefit, but good nutrition is still the key to successful weight control. And, if you work your food and exercise together as a team effort, you'll see even more weight loss results.

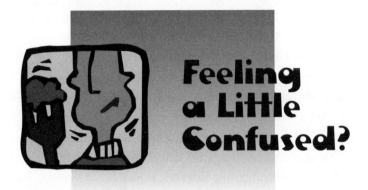

Feeling a Little Confused?

I must tell you, it seems that American teens are just as mixed up about good healthy nutrition as their parents. Maybe the fact that you're always feeling rushed for time and striving for great grades while juggling a ton of after-school activities has eliminated your ability to properly relax and feed yourself. Unfortunately, having too little time with too much to do has created a national population that is more than 66% overweight. Kids have been affected even more than adults have. The average American child is ten pounds heavier than they were only eight years ago and is getting 6% bigger every year...THAT'S STAGGERING!

Only a small percentage of teens are involved in organized sports but, medical studies have also shown that those students who are involved in sports or performance related activities have shown an accelerated rate of eating disorders. The pressure to achieve peak performance and appearance has made this group of teens over-exercise, use unhealthy dieting techniques like vomiting, fasting, diuretics, laxatives and other drugs. The pressure to meet weight goals for sports like wrestling or the desire to look thinner and more attractive, has turned teens to unhealthy and dangerous weight-control alternatives.

I bet you didn't know that kids who are known to repeatedly diet are eight times more likely to develop dangerous eating disorders. This does not have to be you. Eating can be simple when you know what to do.

That's why I want you to look at what you eat along with why you think you are overweight. If we can get to the cause of what you think is your problem, we can solve it.

Kids that aren't exercising or involved in sports during the summer break oftentimes find themselves needing to take desperate action when it comes time to weigh-in for school activities. This doesn't have to be you either. When you're in control, you're in control all of the time. Soon you will find yourself armed with all the information you'll need to make eating and lifestyle adjustments that allow you to stay at your optimum weight and appearance any time of the year.

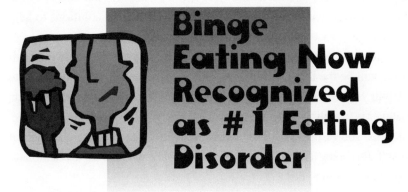

Binge Eating Now Recognized as #1 Eating Disorder

I bet you didn't realize that the #1 eating disorder in America does not deal with eliminating food for weight control through purging like Bulimia, or starvation as in Anorexia. The #1 eating disorder is over-eating or binging.

If you're a stress eater, you may not be entirely aware of it. But, that certainly doesn't mean you're a binger either. A lot of people are emotional eaters. Stress or upset drives many folks straight to the refrigerator. I know...I was a major stress-eater. Show me a problem and I was out chasing an Entenmanns' donut truck! But, there is a very big difference between the person whose occasional depression causes crazy and temporary overeating compared to the person that regularly binges.

The fact is, from a medical point of view, it is impossible to physically be a "stress-eater" because your body's hunger trigger actually shuts down in times of stress. If you're eating when you're upset, it's because you have decided to find comfort in food. The file system in your brain has been programmed to tell you to eat when your emotions fall below the line on your happiness median. Don't misunderstand me, your pattern of turning to food when you need an emotional boost is very real. You have created a belief that food will make you feel better, so it probably does. But, by doing this, you have programmed yourself to actually use food as a reward. Sometimes, just being aware of what you're doing to yourself will go a long way to help you find workable solutions to help you stop.

Take the time to understand what foods are good for you and hopefully, they will be the foods you like to eat. In the long run, it's a lot easier to deal with your emotions directly rather than hide from them behind a pizza. Whatever is troubling you isn't going to go away just by stuffing your face. And, after you're full, you have the additional bonus of being ashamed of yourself for being frustrated enough to grossly overeat as a reaction to what's really eating you!

Whenever you feel frustrated or upset, try and identify the source of the problem. It's certainly possible that what is bothering you may be out of your control when it comes to finding a solution. What you need to do when you're upset is let yourself FEEL the emotions you're feeling and don't try to hold your upset inside. If someone else is responsible for your bad feelings, make them aware. I know that sounds pretty simple and it's not always practical, but 'facing your foes' is oftentimes the best medicine.

If you really think about it, you usually have very little to lose if you tell people how you feel. Sometimes, just by talking about it, you may find that the situation or person you're upset with has a different perspective than you do about the same events. Holding ugly feelings inside (where they can literally eat at you from the inside out), only makes the problem worse than it already is. And turning to the refrigerator or pantry to help you feel better only makes you feel worse than you did before. The problems are still there, and now there is MORE of YOU that needs to deal with them.

If you stick to a few basic rules, it's really not tough to manage your weight. Don't even consider doing anything that is unnatural or doesn't make good health sense. Binge eating, vomiting or failing to eat at all doesn't help you accomplish anything, but it may put you in an early grave. You are on the right track now. Food can be your friend and help you live a long and healthy life. Remember, there is nothing on your "off limits" list when it comes to food. Logically, you may not eat unlimited ice cream and cake but you can certainly have a scoop or a slice once in a while. Keeping this in mind will also help you from feeling deprived. When you're not deprived, your cravings will go away.

If you're not sure whether or not you might be a binge-eater, some of the signs of this eating disorder are:

- Eating large quantities of food alone.
- Feeling a lack of control or inability to stop eating during a binge.
- Post-binge feelings of self-hatred, guilt, depression or disgust.
- Purging, fasting, excessive exercise or other compensation.
- Binge two or more times every week.

If any of these items sound like they might apply to you, you're not alone. Two out of five Americans find themselves binge-eating on a regular basis. This is a much higher percentage than anorexic behavior, which applies to less than 1% of the population, or bulimic actions which affects 1%-3%.

Before you can lose weight effectively, you must face what put the weight on you in the first place. You're going to hear me say that a lot. Denying that you have an eating disorder will not enable you to cure it. Even if your weight condition is not associated with an eating disorder, you must also become aware of the foods and the conditions that cause you so much trouble.

Classic binge-eaters see themselves as failures. They've tried many diets, losing and regaining the same weight again and again. Surveys have shown that nearly one-third of the clients on organized weight loss programs meet the criteria for binge-eating disorder. Over-eating can become an addiction similar to alcoholism or drug use if not detected and resolved. Most binge-eating sufferers say binges are triggered by anger, sadness, boredom, anxiety or some other negative emotion.

If this applies to you, it's important that you recognize the connection between feelings and binge eating episodes in order to break the pattern and overcome the urge. It's wonderful for you to try to work this problem out yourself, but you should share your condition with your parents or even a therapist. Sometimes, it takes looking at your situation from the outside to help you identify the source of the disorder and, once you know what it is, you will be able to work through it much faster and easier.

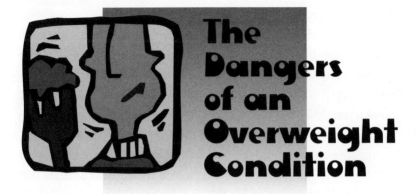

The Dangers of an Overweight Condition

Besides not feeling good or being embarrassed about how you look, there are many statistics that show that an overweight condition can have many negative effects on your health and your body. Most teens feel that these statistics don't apply to them because they think that unhealthy bodies only apply to older people. But, you will be "older" sooner than you think and this is the only body you're going to have. So, you need to start caring for it properly now. It's important that you understand what you could be in for if you don't get a grip on your weight while you can. If you stay heavy as a teen, it can begin a lifetime of physical ailments and complications that are associated with an overweight body.

Let me give you some facts. A 14-year study conducted by Harvard researchers in 1997, found that weight gains of even 11 to 18 pounds in adult life resulted in a 25% greater chance of suffering or dying of a heart attack. The study evaluated the heart related deaths of more than 115,000 middle-aged women and concluded that more than 40% of those women experienced heart attacks due to weight gain.

Every person has an 'ideal body weight', which is determined from a height, sex, age and bone structure calculation. I'm not trying to freak you out, but your chance of death increases as your body weight increases. In other words, if you are much larger than your ideal weight based on your height, sex, age and bone structure, your chance of dying before your time is much greater.

Being underweight is actually more hazardous than being overweight because having too little body fat creates even greater stress and risk to the body than being obese. So, being too skinny won't make you healthier either!

I'm not trying to be morbid talking about death, but I really need you to fully understand how important weight management is. As a guideline, you can suppose that you could die two to three years early for every 10% you are over your 'ideal weight.' Life insurance companies calculate that the chance of death is increased by 25% in people who are only 5%-15% over their ideal weight, but is increased by more than 400% in people who are more than 25% over their ideal weight!

If you are short, you have an even greater concern because you don't have as much body where you can distribute excess fat as a tall person does. Your risk will be greater with the ratio of waist to hip measurement, so it is critical that you stay as close to your 'ideal weight' as possible.

Although heart problems are most commonly associated with an overweight condition, other life-threatening or life-shortening diseases such as cancer, hypertension, gallbladder disease, lung disorders and diabetes are also high risk possibilities. Breast cancer in women, for example, is 38% more common in ladies that are overweight rather than at their ideal weight. Obesity can push the body into a situation where it is no longer able to control blood sugar levels correctly, so that diabetes may develop, requiring regular insulin shots.

What else do you have to look forward to if you allow yourself to stay overweight? How about lower back pain, aggravated arthritic joint problems, flat feet, circulatory problems such as varicose veins and respiratory problems such as shortness of breath, snoring and, particularly in men, gout attacks. Hiatal hernias, which sometimes feels like heartburn can also become a regular occurrence.

The eating habits you establish now can affect you later in life. Eating large quantities of fatty foods containing hydrogenated oils and trans-fatty acids (which I go into more in the "What's a Food Group and

Why You Care" chapter of this book) are more deadly than just being overweight because bad fats create fat deposits in the body which will be released into your circulatory system. This fat release further screws up your body by blocking the metabolism of good fats like essential fatty acids.

There has not been a specific study to prove if overweight people eat more 'bad fats' than people maintaining their ideal weight, but let's just take a guess. It sure seems logical that overweight people most likely eat a lot more 'junk food' and poor nutritional items than people that are careful about what they put into their bodies. We know, for a fact, that fast-food companies have a pretty specific profile on their customers who tend to overeat and order large orders just for themselves. Their profile says that their customer is overweight and mostly male.

Yo-yo dieting, if you don't already know, is when you gain and lose weight over and over again. It creates an increased health risk because making your body gain and lose over and over does not enable your body to stabilize and function properly. An overweight condition increases the strain on your heart that should pretty much go away once the excess weight is lost. But, in the meantime while you're heavy, it may create some damage to your heart. If you continue to gain and lose weight, you may reduce the risk of heart disease when you are closer to your ideal weight, but the ongoing strain and damage to your heart in the process will increase your chance for sudden cardiac death.

Even as a young person you may consider yourself a yo-yo dieter. If that is the case, then it is my goal to get you to break this trend. The best thing you can do for yourself is eat lots of protein and don't worry about calories. Calories are not important in the scheme of things. What you eat is what's most important. Eating 1500 calories every day coming from healthy, balanced food choices is much better for your weight loss efforts than eating 1500 calories in sugar and junk. All calories are NOT created equal!

Dieting is only a temporary solution, so that's why you should not diet anymore. You must eat in the same way while you are losing your weight that you know you can maintain after you have reached your weight goal. Temporary food changes only mean temporary results. You don't need to deprive yourself, you just need to take control.

Why Do People Have So Much Trouble with Weight?

Obesity researchers and nutritionists are at a loss to figure out how to put the brakes on America's weight gain. You're not alone on this topic. Everyone wonders why, even though we're a lot smarter about nutrition and good health, America is fatter than ever.

I think you will find some of the reasons these professionals give are pretty interesting. I have also included some of the reasons the public said they were overweight based on a Gallup poll that was released in January of 2000. Sometimes, when we see a few of our own reasons for being overweight mixed in with the way other people feel, it helps us to realize that our problems aren't so unusual. It helps us to see how necessary it is to stop the excuses and just solve the problem.

Here was the experts' thinking on why we have trouble with weight:

- Portion sizes are out of control. "Biggie" size portions are encouraged by restaurants everywhere.
- New low-fat and no-fat foods give us a false sense of security that actually sabotage our efforts to lose weight.
- New "miracle drugs & pills" raise false hopes when promoting weight loss because they don't help people break bad eating habits.

- People get discouraged if they don't lose all their weight overnight, or begin unreasonable exercise programs that they don't have time to maintain. When they find all the work isn't worth the effort, they would rather stay overweight.
- Most Americans don't exercise. Only 22% of Americans meet at least the minimum exercise guidelines of thirty minutes of moderate activity most days of the week.
- People feel they must give up their favorite foods in order to lose weight. They don't want to recognize that if they're sensible about what they eat, they can eat anything as long as they don't go crazy. People would simply rather eat everything they want.
- Some people hide behind their weight and don't even try to lose. They have convinced themselves that they will probably gain it back anyway, so why bother trying to lose it at all?

Even though a few of the items listed here may apply to you, don't let yourself use any of these excuses to stop yourself from succeeding. When you take responsibility for yourself and how you eat, there is no reason that you can't enjoy the body you want for the rest of your life. It's so great to feel proud of how you look. If eating more cake and cookies than you need keeps you from your goal, is that treat possibly worth it? I don't think so, and neither do you.

chapter seven

Dieting Makes It Worse

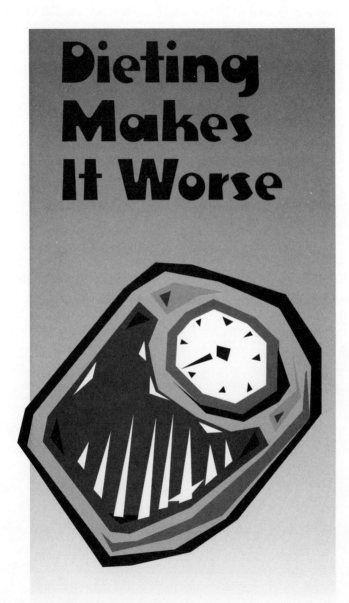

Fad Diets & Weight Problems Go 'Hand-in-Hand'

The problem with fad diets is that they all work - but only temporarily. So it's no wonder that these kinds of diets never die, even though a lot of the time they get exposed by doctors as ineffective, badly balanced nutritionally, or even dangerous.

We have talked about the fact that obesity is a national problem. While nutrition scientists and geneticists probe deeper into causes and cures for obesity, many fat people, as well as those who simply think they are fat, run as fast as they can to find any goofy weight loss program that promises to shed their extra pounds quickly and easily. You can't even turn on the TV without seeing a bunch of infomercials that are full of "lose weight fast", "fat-blocker" type ads. Don't get tricked by all the healthy looking, slim people eating unbelievable desserts and high-fat foods in these commercials. Let's face it...you already know that you can't be thin and load your body up with fat. It's not logical. You may as well learn right now that if something sounds too good to be true in life, it probably is. Weight management needs to be 'manageable' for you. What you're doing right now makes the most sense. You're learning to eat right and understand yourself better in the process. Anything that's worthwhile in life, takes a little effort. If your lifestyle doesn't allow you to weigh and sort food, or carry pre-packaged meals around with you, then diets associated with those practices won't work for you long-term either. What you're doing now makes the most sense. In reading this book, you're learning to eat right and understand yourself better in the process.

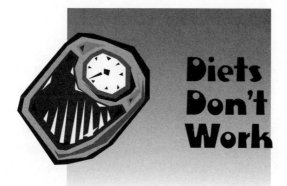

Diets Don't Work

As tempted as you may be to be super good about trying to follow the rules for this program, I can't urge you enough...DON'T DIET! Don't try and make any food changes that are too hard for you or that you can't maintain. It's not realistic to say "I'll never have pizza again." So, don't say it!

Losing weight is all about getting your metabolism fired-up and cooking. The metabolism is your body's system for creating energy and burning up fat. This can't be achieved by starving yourself so, get it straight...you must eat in order to lose weight. In fact, starvation slows metabolic levels even more and ultimately leads to a higher body fat content which is hardly what you need now. When your body doesn't receive the nutrition it requires, it stores fat. So, if you really want to achieve your weight loss goal, it's time to stop dieting and start eating.

First, eat regular meals. Try not to get yourself worked into a starvation frenzy just before meal time because it will only encourage you to eat more. If you eat well-balanced, regular meals throughout the day, your body will use the foods you're eating better.

Second, eat the right balance. Focus on protein first. Fish, chicken, turkey and lean red meats should be the biggest part of each meal. Try to eat at least 10 ounces of some sort of protein daily - that's about three chicken breasts. Protein not only provides all the good stuff that your major organs need, it actually burns itself off during the digestive process. In other words, thirty percent of the protein you eat will actually be eliminated all by itself just by working itself through the digestive system.

You can have all the fruits and vegetables you want so use these foods as snack items, too. Dairy should be limited to one meal each day. For example, if you are having eggs for breakfast, don't have a cheese sandwich for lunch. Keep your starchy carbohydrates down to two or three servings every day. Starches include pasta, rice, potato, corn, breads and cereals. Instead of having any of these items as a main meal, have them as a side dish so you will eat less of them. If you can get out of the habit of eating sandwiches, then that's all the better, too. It's not what's in the sandwich that's a problem, it's the bread. I personally don't like to eat any bread when it's not really "worth it," and I consider two slices of plain bread wrapped around a bunch of meat not "worth it."

Carbohydrates and starches like potato and pasta are converted to sugar in the body for processing, so any unused carbs that you're eating every day will ultimately turn into fat. It takes the body fifteen minutes of jogging just to get rid of a single slice of bread! Think of all the exercise you will need to do each day if you decide to have pancakes for breakfast, a sub-sandwich for lunch and spaghetti for dinner. Even if you eat only fat-free carbohydrates, your body will become a fat-manufacturing machine and your pant size will only increase.

Third, rotate your food - and that doesn't mean just turn your plate around! Don't eat the same things all the time. We are all creatures of habit, but try to eat different foods every day. If you eat chicken Monday, have turkey or roast beef Tuesday. The same rule applies to fruits, vegetables and even spices. If you have a salad made of iceberg lettuce one day, have romaine or bibb lettuce the next. You may not know what all your options are right now, but you will soon. The market is full of lots of different kinds of everything! Learn about all the choices available to you, and when it comes to food, experiment. Retraining your tastebuds to like different and healthier things can be a really fun experience.

Drink water! Water is the only thing that flushes fat out of your body so be sure and drink 6-8, eight ounce glasses of water every day. If you have trouble drinking enough water, drink through a straw. You will find that you will drink two to three times more liquid with each sip when a straw is used. Refillable sport bottles are your best bet to keep track of the water you're drinking. They travel well and usually hold about 32 ounces of liquid. You'll know that you got all of your water in for the day when you drink all the water you've put into two sport bottles.

If you eat like you're on a 'diet,' and return to eating "normally" once you reach your weight goal, you will immediately begin to regain all those unwanted pounds and inches you worked so hard to eliminate. So, don't even THINK about dieting. This is a program you'll do forever...not just for the moment. This isn't a weight management fad that you'll grow out of. It's a way of life.

Don't deny yourself from having any of your favorite foods. Eat smart. You control your eating, don't let your eating control you. You can eat anything - just don't keep eating a bunch of high fat or sugar foods that contain empty calories with little or no nutritional value. When you find the right balance of food for your body, your body's weight will respond pretty quickly. And, the best part is, the better you make yourself eat, the easier it is to eat better! That's right. When your body gets used to healthy, balanced meals, it begins to crave and actually prefer healthy and balanced food items. You will be surprised at how you will begin to crave things that are good for you and how easily you will be able to turn down sugary treats that used to be the things you reached for or ordered first. Once you recognize this change in your eating habits, a lot of the fear you may have about "giving up" certain foods will go away. The stronger you THINK you are, the stronger you WILL BE. Remember, your body believes what YOU believe. When you believe you are in control....YOU ARE!

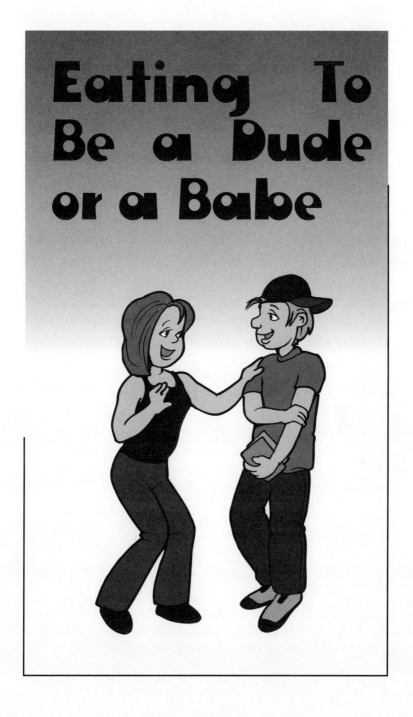

chapter eight

Eating To Be a Dude or a Babe

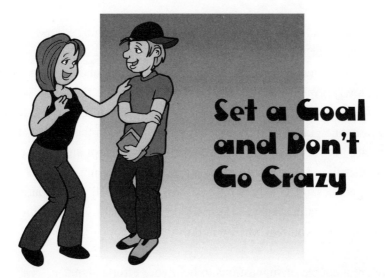

Set a Goal and Don't Go Crazy

Here we go. The best way to start any weight loss program is to set a realistic goal for yourself and don't make a lot of eating changes right away. If you need to lose a lot of weight, do it a little bit at a time. Set a lower goal first so you can see your progress and feel comfortable that this time, you'll get your extra weight off for good. When I had 85 pounds to lose, it seemed like it would take forever before I could imagine all that weight gone. Instead of being excited about each pound I lost, I kept thinking about how much farther I still had to go.

When you set your goals in steps, it's a lot easier to stay motivated and be proud of every pound you've lost along the way. Keep reminding yourself that you didn't gain your weight overnight, you can't expect to lose it overnight either. And I certainly don't want you to get yourself too upset about how long it may take to get thinner, because then you may find yourself in a depression that could cause you to eat. Everything you do should help you to keep your emotional comfort zone above-the-line!

Another tip for keeping your mind in a happy-mode is to stay off the scale. Don't weigh yourself too often. When you do decide to weigh-in, do it at the same time each day so your body is consistently comparing itself under the same conditions. Mornings are best because you are lightest then and have an empty stomach. By weighing yourself at the same time, your measurement will be more accurate.

Instead of making major changes in your eating and lifestyle habits, do it slowly. When you try and do too much at one time, you will get overwhelmed and feel like the effort you are putting into trying to lose weight is one giant and difficult chore. Cut down on the foods that you know are not very good for you. Sweets & candy, chips and pizza can all be on that list. Make an effort to eat more balanced meals full of meats and vegetables. You'll be surprised how easy it will be to continually improve your eating habits. Before long, you'll get used to eating right and prefer how you feel when you do!

Here are a couple of suggestions to help your efforts along:

- Eat at home more often. Studies show that we tend to eat larger quantities and fattier foods when we eat out.

- Put down your fork between bites. Don't be in such a hurry to finish your meal.

- Don't eat a lot of 'fat-free' products thinking you're eating less calories. Fat-free bread, pasta and stuff actually manufacture fat in the body if you're not burning them up!

- Make choices. Have one "naughty" choice per day rather than a lot of them. If you'd like dessert after dinner, don't have ice cream at lunchtime.

- Try to eat the majority of your meals before 5:00 PM so you're not going to sleep with a full stomach.

- Add more beta-carotene and vitamin C to your diet by substituting sweet potatoes for regular baked potatoes. Not only are they better for you, we tend to eat sweet potatoes with less butter and no sour cream or bacon.

- If you must have meat on your pizza, use Canadian bacon instead of pepperoni or sausage. Cheese-less pizza is also good with the right sauce and a little parmesan instead.

- Drink skim, 1% or 2% milk instead of whole milk whenever possible. This is especially easy if you eat cereal because the flavor of the milk is hidden in the flavor of the cereal.

- Put smaller portions on your plate, then come back for more if you're still hungry. Most people try to eat everything on their plate even when they're full. Less quantity on the plate puts less pressure on you.

- Eat when you're hungry and stop when you're full. Don't allow yourself to be overly hungry or starving before you eat and once your stomach feels satisfied that you've eaten enough...STOP!

- If you find that you're eating too many snacks, eat more protein during mealtime so that you will not get as hungry throughout the day. Protein burns more fat, so by eating more of it, your food begins to work for you and not against you!

- Try mini-meals. Eat small quantities of food more often throughout the day so you never get too hungry.

- Drink water. Remember, water is the only way to flush fats from your body.

- Don't deny yourself any favorites. Try to take a taste of the things you'd really like to eat so you don't create cravings that are difficult to control later.

- Don't eat in front of the TV. Studies have shown that when people are distracted, they tend to eat more.

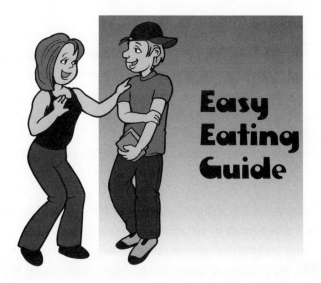

Easy Eating Guide

Learning to eat right in order to help you to lose weight doesn't have to be painful and it doesn't need to take forever. Don't go crazy and plan everything you put in your mouth. This only creates a focus on food that we're trying to eliminate. You want to make reasonable changes that are not that big a deal to you, so you can live with your changes for the rest of your life. I can't stress enough that temporary food changes only mean temporary weight loss. Be responsible for what you decide to eat and don't eat things you know are not good for you.

We've already talked about how denying yourself only starts you craving the food you're trying to ignore. I think you'll agree with me when I say, "we always want what we can't have"- so feel comfortable that everything you could possibly want to put into your mouth is on your "can have" list...but, within reason.

In the very near future, what is going to surprise you most, is that you won't really ever think about many of the items you crave all the time now. Just like your body, your taste buds are triggered by your brain's memory. Soon you will begin to crave foods that are good for you and you'll never miss the unhealthy stuff you think you can't live without.

I am a believer in eating by category - not calorie counting, or weighing out portions. When it comes to how much you can eat, I want you to set your own personal portion limits that are logical for you.

Obviously, if you decide to eat "biggie," oversized portions, you are not acting in the best interests of your weight loss efforts and you'll need to take responsibility for those bad choices. If you don't see the weight loss results you're looking for after pretending that giant portions are OK for you, don't blame the program - look to some false beliefs you may have developed that are really only wishful thinking!

Follow these few food guideline tips and weight control is not far behind:

- Eat as much protein (chicken, seafood, turkey, lean red meat) as you can - a minimum of 10 ounces every day is best.
- Fruits and vegetables are unlimited daily. Keep high sugar fruits like watermelon, pineapple, and bananas limited to three times per week. Citrus fruits like oranges, grapefruit, lemons, as well as apples, cantaloupe and a handful of berries can all be eaten every day.
- Select 1 meal to eat from your dairy category. This will help you to control your fat intake. If you have eggs for breakfast, don't have cheese for lunch. Consider 1 glass of low-fat milk as a free bee: It can be used on your cereal.
- Eat 2 portions of carbohydrates each day such as rice, pasta, potato, corn, cereal or bread. For example, you could select a sandwich for lunch & a potato or pasta side dish for dinner. Eat sweet potato over regular potatoes whenever you can. They are much better for you and they don't require all the butter, sour cream and condments to make them taste good.
- Drink lots of water.

Don't make yourself crazy when it comes to serving sizes for starches like breads, pasta, rice, cereal, etc. Each person has their own individual serving size in mind. Whatever you consider a serving to be is a serving size for YOU. In other words, if you are currently eating 6 servings of carbs every day, you can still eat 2 of those current servings, no matter what size those servings are - just stop eating the extra 4. The outrageous example I usually use is my "loaf of bread" example: If you think of a whole loaf of bread as being one serving (yes, I already know that's ridiculous but stick with me on this!) and you are now eating six loaves of bread every day, isn't it reasonable to think that you will lose weight if you only eat two loaves now and stop eating four? Anybody who cuts four loaves of bread out of their diet every day can't help but lose weight. See what I mean?

Don't be concerned with the size of your fruit, vegetable or protein portions. Just make sure you eat a balance of food daily. The less complicated you make your weight loss program, the easier it will be to follow and the more successful it will be for you.

Now let's talk about what I call my "worth it" foods. Whenever you think about eating something with questionable food value or high fat content, at least be sure it's "worth it." Eating a piece of bread "just because it's there" does not fall into my 'worth it' category. To be 'worth it,' it would have to be wonderfully delicious.

Here's a recap of five easy-to-follow steps that will get you well on your way to the "dude or babe" body you're looking for:

1. **Stop Dieting and Eat Realistically.** Don't make drastic food changes that you can't maintain forever. You must take an honest look at what you eat and how you eat and evaluate your problem food areas. Sweets, cheeses and snack foods are obvious areas that you will most likely need to deal with. There isn't any advantage to eliminating items from your daily menu while trying to lose weight if you already know you're going to go back to eating those items once you have reached your weight loss goal.

2. **Have Food Variety.** This is the single biggest thing you can do every day to effect your body's metabolism. Even if you didn't change one thing in your regular diet and never ate the same things two days in a row, you would see your weight go down. If you eat the same foods every day, and most of us do, you're slowing down your metabolism by putting it into a regular pattern.

Try to eat different foods every 24 hours. If you eat chicken on Monday, don't have it again until Wednesday. This rule applies to everything you eat, even if those things don't have any calories. Lettuce is an excellent example. If you eat iceberg lettuce on Monday, have bibb lettuce on Tuesday and romaine on Wednesday.

The change will keep your metabolic level much more active and your body functioning more efficiently.

3. **Drink Water.** Water is the only liquid you can drink that will flush fats out of your body. Water beverages such as coffee or tea are not water. Soda is not water. You need to drink six to eight 8-ounce glasses of water every day to get rid of the fats your body is breaking down. If you don't like water, try some of the flavored waters now available like Syfo or Perrier. Make sure your mom checks the label before she buys bottled water for you. Be sure the label says "O calories." A lot of "water beverages" have as many or even more calories than soda and are not water even though the label clearly says "water beverage." And, don't for get to drink through a strawand not just from the glass. You will drink two to three times more water if you drink through a straw. Even though that seems dumb, it's true.

4. **Food Trading.** There are always a lot of options when it comes to finding better food choices. Once you start to find alternative foods that satisfy your tastebuds but have less fat and more protein in them, it is a lot easier to make smart choices.

Here's a couple of hints: Grate your cheese. Don't slice it and you will trick your mind into thinking you are eating a larger quantity. Try eating turkey bacon instead of pork bacon. Eat sugar-free popsicles or fat-free frozen yogurt instead of ice cream. Eat fat-free pretzels not chips. At any level, for any kind of food category, there is an alternative that tastes good and is better for you.

5. **Eat What You Crave.** This is probably the most important step. No matter what food item you crave, be sure to include a serving or two of it for the week. It's true that you can't live on chocolate cake, but you can plan on having it once or twice a week to give yourself a treat to look forward to. Soon you'll start to develop an eating plan that allows you all the things you like regularly, not necessarily every day, and then all you need to do is to maintain that same plan forever. If you deny yourself your favorite foods, you will eventually begin to binge on those items until you have satisfied your body's craving.

Be realistic about what you can and can't live with. This is true of what you eat and also how active you think you can be. If you are like the majority of Americans who don't like to exercise, your diet must consist of high protein foods like chicken, seafood and lean red meats rather than lots of carbohydrates such as bread, pasta, rice or potato.

Without doing a lot of exercise, you have no way to burn off the sugar that unused carbohydrates create when they create energy in your body. That sugar, or glucose, is what your body will ultimately turn into fat. I already told you that it takes fifteen minutes of jogging for your body to burn off a single slice of bread, so you need to keep your carbs low if you have a low activity level.

Be smart and think thin. Fill up on lean meats, fruits and vegetables and keep your dairy and starch intake to one or two servings a day. Medical experts feel that weight loss is fifty percent physical and fifty percent psychological. Maintain a positive attitude, exercise and create a realistic eating program you can live with forever.

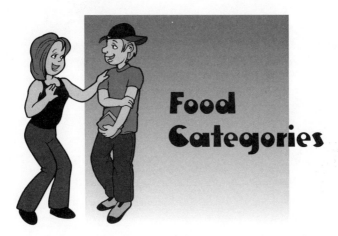

Food Categories

Eating and meal planning shouldn't have to take up your day when you learn to eat by category. On the next three pages is a list of foods in each of the food groups so you can see how easy it is to understand the options you have. If a food is not listed, it does not mean that it should be avoided. I have covered only the basics here.

PROTEIN - at least 10 ounces daily

LOW-FAT PROTEIN - unlimited daily

HIGH-FAT PROTEIN - 3 times per week

VEGETABLES - unlimited daily

LOW-SUGAR FRUITS - unlimited daily

HIGHER SUGAR FRUITS - 3 times per week

DAIRY - 1 serving daily

STARCHES - 2 servings daily

WATER - 8 eight ounce glasses daily

•Choose Low-Fat Foods Whenever Possible•

Menu Guide

PROTEIN

Seafood: Low-Fat
Unlimited
Cod
Crab
Dolphin
Flounder
Grouper
Haddock
Halibut
Lobster
Salmon
Scallops
Scrod
Sole
Shrimp
Swordfish
Tuna Fish (water packed)
Whitefish

Meat - Low Fat
Unlimited
Beef/Chicken or Calves
Liver
Chicken Breast
Turkey Breast

Vegetarian Protein
Limited
Boca Burgers®
Tofu
Soy Milk
Veggie Burgers

Meat - Higher Fat
3x Per Week (If Desired)
Club Steak
Flank Steak
Filet Mignon
Ground Turkey
Ground Sirloin (Hamburger)
Lamb Chops
London Broil
Pork Chops
Roast Beef
Round Steak
Veal Chops
Veal Cutlet
Veal Rump

Menu Guide

Dairy (Fats)
1 Serving Daily
Butter
Cheese
Cream Cheese
Cottage Cheese
Eggs
Mayonnaise
Milk
Parmesan Cheese
Yogurt

Vegetables - Unlimited
Asparagus
Bean Sprouts
Broccoli
Cabbage
Carrots
Celery
Cucumbers
Eggplant
Green Beans
Lettuce
Mushrooms
Mustard Greens
Onions
Peppers
Radishes

Spinach
Squash
Tomatoes
Zucchini

Fruits - Low-Sugar
Unlimited
Apples
Cantaloupe
Grapefruit
Oranges

Fruits - Higher Sugar
3x Per Week If Desired
Apricots
Bananas
Cherries
Grapes
Honeydew
Papaya
Pear
Pineapple
Plums
Tangerine
Watermelon

Menu Guide

STARCHES
2 Servings Daily
Bread
Bagel (scooped)
Cereal (hot or cold)
Crackers
Corn
Pancakes/Waffles
Pasta
Peas
Pita
Potato
Rice
Tortillas

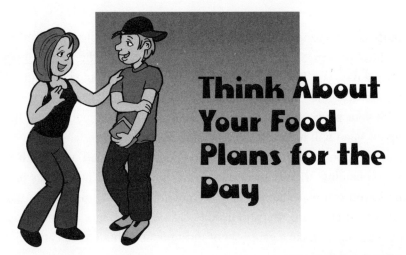

Think About Your Food Plans for the Day

When I started BioDietetics, formerly Fit America, in 1992, I wanted to create a nice and easy way to eat that anyone could follow. Even though my guidelines are very simple, they are also pretty specific and the kids I work with find them pretty sensible and easy too. If you don't eat enough protein for example, the program will not be nearly as successful.

It is a proven fact that people who have detailed guidelines to follow, even the most simple guidelines, will do better than people who feel that they really don't know how to make all of their own decisions when it comes to thinking about what to eat. When you learn to eat by category, and not get caught up with weighing, measuring and portioning out your food, maintaining good eating patterns will become an easy part of your life. You are now reprogramming yourself to prefer feeling better and eating better. Stick with it!

If you try to lose weight just by eating less, you're going to fail. When you try and stop yourself from eating the foods you love, it encourages binge eating - so that option's out, too. If you stick to my eating guidelines when you're thinking about what you want to eat, you can't go wrong.

When you know ahead of time that you have a sporting event at school and everyone will probably go for pizza afterward, don't have any other carbs during the day and save all your starch allowance for pizza night. Since pizza is not going to give your body all the protein it needs for the day, you'll want to be sure to eat chicken or some other source of protein for your other two meals. It's also a good idea to order a salad with your pizza. Not only are the green vegetables good for you, filling up on salad will help you to eat less of the fattier pizza.

You don't need to feel like you should get carried away with your meal planning. If you know ahead of time about special lunches or dinners, you can plan the rest of your day around those meals. No matter what your plans are, you still need to eat a balanced mix of food throughout each day. Make a game out of meal planning until good eating habits replace old, bad ones.

No matter what anyone tells you, feel confident that you can make up tomorrow for any "food mistakes" you may have made today. Just don't make over-doing it a regular practice. If you find you ate too many starches on Monday, eat little or no starches on Tuesday. I never want you to feel that "a bad food day" messed up your weight loss efforts to the point that you might as well give up. Every "good food day" is a successful one. It's successful for your body and it shows that you are capable of personal success too. We all have "bad food days." It's not the end of the world...it's just the beginning of a new, 'good food day' for you!

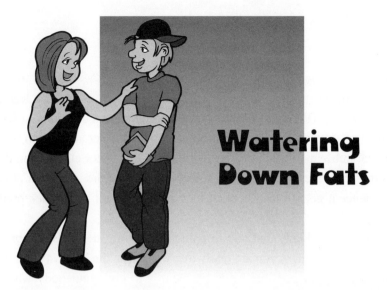

Watering Down Fats

Losing fat is a lot easier than you think. Just drink water! I'm not kidding!

Here's one that will surprise you...incredible as it may seem, water is quite possibly the single most important thing you can do for losing weight and keeping it off. Although most of us take it for granted, water may be the only true "magic potion" for permanent weight loss. It's certainly the easiest.

Water helps suppress the appetite naturally so you're not hungry. It also helps the body metabolize stored fat which means water helps break fat down and flush it out. Studies have shown that when people don't drink enough water, the body will have more fat deposits causing people to actually gain weight.

Here's why: The kidneys can't function properly without enough water. When the kidneys aren't working right, some of what they should be doing is dumped into the liver to be processed. One of the liver's primary functions is to metabolize stored fat into usable energy for the body. But, if the liver has to do some of the kidneys' work, it can't operate at full throttle. As a result, it metabolizes less fat, and more fat remains stored in the body so weight loss stops.

Drinking enough water is the best treatment for people who tend to hold fluids. When the body gets less water, it sees it as a threat to survival and begins to hold onto every drop which can consequently lead to swollen limbs. Diuretics, which are water-reducing medications, offer a short-lived solution at best. They force out stored water along with some essential nutrients. Again, the body thinks all this water elimination that is going on inside of you is a threat and will replace the lost water at the first chance it gets so the 'swollen foot' condition will come back pretty fast.

It isn't very likely that you're going to have a water retention problem at your age unless you are really overweight, so the best way to overcome any kind of possible water problem is to give your body what it needs: plenty of water. Eating a lot of salt may also be the reason that your hands or feet swell. Your body can only use a limited amount of salt. The more salty foods you eat, the more water your system hangs onto in order to dilute it. If you think you have a "sweet tooth" problem, eating a lot of salty stuff may also be part of the reason. Using a lot of salt on your food or eating food that contains a lot of salt already will usually make your body crave more sweets. Isn't that weird? I guess the bottom line is: Don't over-do the salt OR the sweets!

Since we know that water is the key to losing fat, it makes sense that an overweight person needs more water than a thin one.

Water also helps to maintain proper muscle tone by giving muscles their natural ability to contract, and it prevents dehydration. It also helps to prevent sagging skin that usually follows after a lot of weight loss.

The water you drink stays pretty busy working all over your body. It does something just about everywhere! While water is flushing out fats, it's also flushing out toxins...the same toxins that can cause acne or other skin outbreaks. Shrinking cells are fattened up by water, which plumps the skin and leaves it clear, healthy and resilient. See, your face can benefit, too!

Water helps rid the body of waste and, during weight loss time, the body has a lot more waste to get rid of. All metabolized fat that has been broken down and is ready to be flushed away must be eliminated from the body through urine. Water will also help relieve constipation if you're having a tough time going to the bathroom.

As you have just learned, water is important for a bundle of reasons. Here again are a few basic true facts about water:

- The body will not function properly without enough water.
- Your body cannot get rid of unwanted, metabolized fat without enough water.
- Water that stays in the body shows up as excess weight.
- To get rid of excess water you must drink MORE water!
- Drinking water is essential to weight loss...it's the only way to flush fat from the body.

Now, the next question..."How much water is enough?" On the average, a person should drink six to eight 8-ounce glasses every day. That is about two quarts. If you are really overweight, you need one additional glass for every 25 pounds of excess weight you carry around with you. The amount of water you drink should also be increased if you are exercising, or if you spend a lot of time outside where the weather is hot and dry.

Cold water is absorbed into the system more quickly than warm water. It also tastes a lot better. If you're not crazy about the flavor of water and that's why it's hard for you to drink, add a squeeze of lemon or lime. And, don't forget to drink water through a straw so you can actually drink two to three times more than you can when you drink from a glass.

YOU MAY BE DEHYDRATED AND NOT EVEN KNOW IT! If your skin is itchy and dry, or you're tired all the time and suffer from headaches, you could be depriving yourself of water to the point of dehydration which is a fancy way of saying your body is "all dried out."

Drinking soda products or juice doesn't provide the body with the water it needs to operate as well as it should, or get rid of the excess fat you want to see go away. When you consider that water makes up about 70% of the body's solid tissue, helps regulate temperature, carries nutrients and oxygen to cells, removes waste, cushions joints and protects organs and tissues, that jumbo diet cola doesn't look so good.

A great way to know if your body needs water is thirst. If you're thirsty, you're already about two glasses behind in your body's water needs for the day so...DRINK UP!

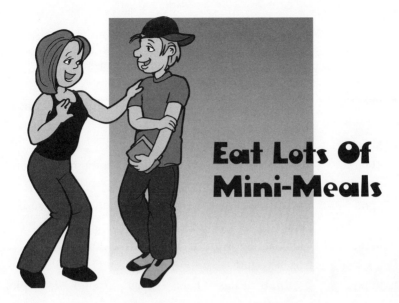

Eat Lots Of Mini-Meals

Whenever you can, try and eat small meals throughout the day and not try to get a whole day's worth of nourishment and food all at one time. Mini-meals are not snacks, but might make it easier for you to keep control while not ever feeling really hungry. You're still going to eat healthy stuff, you're just breaking your meals down into smaller portions this way. And when you eat small meals throughout the day, it can actually help you to lose weight faster.

It's a lot easier for the body to process small amounts of food rather than trying to process big ones. Eating smaller amounts of food throughout the day will also help keep your metabolism more active. Since raising the metabolism is the key to weight loss, try not to eat large quantities of food all at one time.

Include some source of protein at each mini-meal if possible, and vary your vegetable, fruit and carbohydrate selections. Keep in mind that eating a balanced diet doesn't mean eating from all the food groups at every meal. It means that you eat from all the food groups at some time every day.

Let me give you a few examples of one day's mini-meals:

7:30 am:	2 scrambled eggs , turkey bacon, 1 slice whole wheat toast
10:00 am:	Handful of blueberries
12:30 pm:	1/2 Turkey Sandwich with tomato & lettuce 1 apple
3:00 pm:	Cantaloupe with 1/2 cup cottage cheese or yogurt
6:30 pm:	Chicken filet w/green salad and 1/2 cup rice and 1/2 cup frozen yogurt
8:30 pm:	2 thick Roast beef slices around 1/4 pickle w/ mustard
10:00 pm:	Raw vegetables with light ranch dressing

Balance in your daily food selections is very important. You want to have a combination of proteins, fruits, vegetables, starches and dairy products every day. For some, eating little meals like fruit or sliced meats can help make the bulk of their menus quick and handy. But, even though fruit is excellent for you, it doesn't give your body all the proper nutrition it needs all by itself. It is also high in natural sugar. So, keep roasted or barbecued chicken, sliced turkey from a roasted bird (not processed deli meat) and roast beef slices handy. They are all great for you and easy to grab as a quick snack.

You don't need to create a formal menu for the day, but, think ahead about where you'll be for each meal so you'll know what you might be eating and then you can plan around that. Mini-meals just give you another path on your new road to self-control!

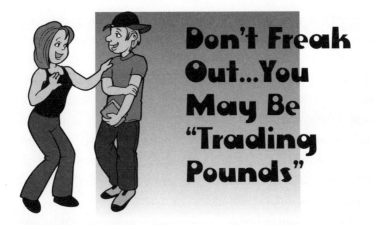

Don't Freak Out...You May Be "Trading Pounds"

When the scale goes down or you feel that your clothes are fitting better, you'll know you're losing weight. Either of these happy moments means you have lost inches as well as pounds. But, don't be surprised if you see that you're getting smaller all over without a pound change when you step on the scale. You're still losing weight but you may be 'trading pounds.' Just for the record, trading pounds is a good thing!

Fat is lighter than muscle, so one pound of fat takes up much more space on your body than one pound of muscle. I'm going to use ball sizes just to better illustrate my point. A pound of fat may be the size of a tennis ball and a pound of muscle may be the size of a golf ball. When you eat a lot of protein, you are building lean muscle mass, which is good. If you lose one pound of fat at the same time you build one pound of lean muscle mass, you may not see the scale move but you will be smaller in size. In effect, you have traded the tennis ball for the golf ball and the golf ball is smaller. That's what I mean by 'trading pounds.' Even though you may not have lost pounds when you step on a scale, your overall body fat percentage has gone down causing you to drop inches.

Most people find that they are eating more protein with this program than they have ever eaten before. I also want to point out that they are eating better and healthier than ever before, too. But, they are still eating more. Lean muscle mass weighs five times more than fat for the same physical size so, as your body becomes leaner, it may actually become heavier.

Some of the people I have worked with have told me that they went from a 37% body fat level to as low as 17%. They tell me they are physically thinner and leaner, but they are now heavier than they were when they had been at this same body size before. Don't be surprised if you see a drastic reduction in inches before the scale moves down as much as you'd like. It does not mean you aren't losing. You'll know that you're losing because your clothing will fit much better.

There is a supplement that I would encourage you to take - I am a firm believer of essential fatty acid (EFA) supplements. Essential fatty acids are the good fats your body needs to operate efficiently. Your body cannot be completely fat-free or it will die. All your major organs are lubricated with essential fats. But, when the body is deficient in EFAs, it will store body fat and not let it go. Taking EFA's will help your body eliminate bad fat without messing with the rest of your organ functions. If you're going to take an essential fatty acid supplement, be sure that the one you select is formulated for weight loss and not body-building.

Just to be sure you're really losing weight and not just fooling yourself when the scale doesn't show it, measure your waist & hips and keep a record of the inches you've lost. If you don't want to use a tape measure because the actual measurement may be too depressing, use a ribbon. Wrap the ribbon around your waist and cut it at the exact point where the two ends meet. Once a week, wrap the ribbon around your waist at the same location you measured the first time and see how much of the two ends overlap. Mark the overlap with a pen so you can watch your progress and see how well you're doing.

Remember, if you're eating a whole lot more protein than you've been eating in the past, the rebuilding of your body's muscles will not show on the scale but it will show on you.

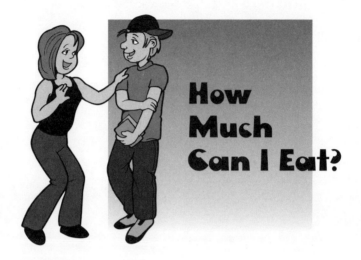

How Much Can I Eat?

"How much can I eat?" is a tough question and unfortunately, I don't have a specific answer. I'm not trying to avoid something I know you want to know but, everyone is an individual when it comes to figuring out how much food their body needs. Since you're not going to diet, you can eat anything. That means, as you start to learn what foods are good for you, you'll try to eat more of those. When you know that you can have any of your favorite foods you want (within reason!), then you will have no need to crave and binge on items that will mess up your weight loss efforts.

For the most part, you're now eating by food group during the day. I don't want you to count calories or weigh portions. I know I keep bringing this up, but I really want to drive my point home. I have found that planning and weighing and sorting out food makes people think about what they're eating all the time. It actually creates a preoccupation with food that, quite frankly, I'm trying to help you grow out of. There's a big difference between thinking about your day so you can make a 'game-plan' for your eating and constantly thinking about every little thing you put into your mouth. Don't make yourself crazy with this... just make smart choices and eat.

When it comes to serving sizes, these are individual too. A serving size for one person may be quite different for another. My daughter used to eat a bowl of cereal in the morning filled to the top in a serving dish that I could put enough mashed potatoes in to serve four people! My son liked to eat his cereal out of a coffee mug. Obviously, both of them considered themselves to have eaten "a single serving."

When I say you can have two servings of starch daily, that means you can have two of the portion sizes you consider to be a "normal" size for you. You may now be thinking that your concept of portion size is what caused your weight problem in the first place and, since that may be true, let me give you an example of what I mean so you don't continue to overeat. I'm going to use my ridiculous bread example again because it gives you the right mental image.

Let's pretend you used to eat six servings of bread throughout the day and you considered an entire loaf of bread to be a serving. My food group menu guide says you can only eat two servings of bread each day. If you reduce the amount of bread you eat from six loaves to two loaves, you have eliminated four loaves of bread from your diet every day. I am sure you can see that you will be able to successfully lose weight if you cut the amount of carbohydrates you're eating by four loaves of bread each and every day.

Even though this is an extreme example, it's the best example I know to show you how relatively unimportant a portion size is. What is important is to make sure that you are not increasing the size of your two servings by changing your belief of what you call a serving size. Be sure you don't make your new serving size the equivalent of the six you used to eat before!

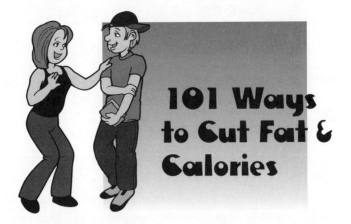

101 Ways to Cut Fat & Calories

Eating better and cutting fats way down doesn't have to be tough. There are a lot of ways that you can cut back on fat without giving up taste or making any radical changes. Sometimes, you just need to know HOW. So, try this:

AT BREAKFAST

1. Instead of regular syrup on pancakes, French toast or waffles, use 2 tablespoons of light syrup, jelly or crushed berries.

2. Top pancakes and oatmeal with fresh fruit or applesauce instead of butter.

3. Use lowfat cottage cheese, jelly or spreadable fruit instead of butter on bread or toast.

4. Eat fat-free breakfast bars or buy bars made with rice instead of granola.

5. Cook omelets with egg whites or egg substitutes.

6. Include vegetables like peppers or broccoli in omelets to replace cheese. If you use cheese, grate a small amount of sharp cheddar to give your food a nice cheese taste.

7. Cook in non-stick pan or use fat-free cooking spray.

8. Make cinnamon toast on 40-calorie bread instead of using French bread.

9. Eat Canadian bacon instead of regular bacon.

10. Beware of oversized bagels - eat bialys instead.

11. Try nonfat or low-fat yogurt with crunchy cereal instead of granola.

12. Sweeten unsweetened cereal with fresh berries or sugar substitute.

13. Drink 1%, 2% or skim milk.

14. Don't eat oversized portions like mega-muffins.

LIGHT LUNCHES

15. Eat raw vegetables rather than veggies marinated in oil when eating at salad bars.

16. Make tuna or chicken salad with light mayonnaise, mustard or non-fat yogurt.

17. Lend the flavor of cheese to salads, tacos and pastas by grating small amounts on top. Use hard cheeses rather then soft ones - hard cheese has less fat.

18. Make your own salad dressings with balsamic vinegar, mustard and herbs.

19. When ordering a Caesar salad, eliminate the croutons.

20. Always get dressing on the side then dip the fork in before stabbing each bite.

21. Use salsa instead of dressings for salads and veggie sandwiches.

22. Don't add breadstuffs to salads.

23. Eat sandwiches on light bread or pita pockets rather than croissants or rolls.

24. Use mustard not mayonnaise.

25. Make sandwiches heavy on the meat, light on cheese.

26. Buy low-fat frozen yogurt instead of ice cream.

27. Eat fresh cold cuts from the butcher section not processed meats or bologna.

DINING OUT

28. To ease bread basket temptation, take one piece and tear off bite-sized pieces.

29. Order an appetizer as an entrée at restaurants that serve large portions.

30. Share your entrée with your dinner companion and order extra salads.

31. Order food a la carte instead of all-you-can-eat type buffets.

32. Choose clear soups instead of cream-based soups.

33. Order pizza with lots of veggies and light on the cheese.

34. Eat a sweet potato or rice instead of fries.

35. Order pasta with tomato sauce instead of cream sauces.

36. Drain oily sauce from Chinese food by serving portions with a fork or chopstix.

37. Have fish, chicken or meats broiled, baked, steamed or roasted, not fried or creamed.

38. Try to eat light meat poultry over dark meat.

39. Select lean cuts of beef such as London broil, round steak or roasts.

40. Trim visible fat or skin from meat & poultry.

41. Eat fish and skinless poultry more often than red meat.

42. Use cocktail sauce or lemon juice not tarter sauce on fish.

43. Order one dessert for all to share.

44. Have cappuccino and other coffee-based drinks made with skim milk.

HOME COOKING

45. Bake breaded chicken and fish on a non-stick baking pan in the oven instead of frying.

46. Sauté foods in chicken or vegetable stock, or tomato juice instead of oil or butter.

47. Keep olive oil in a spray bottle to lightly coat sauté pans.

48. Grill, bake or roast your meat, poultry and fish.

49. Skip the gravy. Use mustard or unsweetened applesauce on roasted birds.

50. Make your own taco shells by hanging soft tortillas directly over racks and baking at 400° until crisp.

51. Make a grilled cheese sandwich by grating 1-1/2 tablespoons of low-fat cheese on the bread instead of using American cheese.

52. Refrigerate homemade soups overnight then spoon off the fat before reheating.

53. Replace side dishes of macaroni and potato salad with lighter fare like carrot or cabbage salads made with vinegar instead of mayonnaise.

54. Make your favorite dips with nonfat yogurt or creamed cottage cheese instead of sour cream or butter.

55. Flavor mashed potatoes with nonfat yogurt and herbs instead of sour cream.

56. Make your own French fries by cutting 1/4 inch slices of potato then sprinkle with paprika or salt and bake at 350° for 35 to 40 minutes. Turn once.

57. Spruce up baked potatoes with plain, nonfat yogurt or cottage cheese mixed with chives.

58. Bake or microwave a sweet potato and sprinkle with cinnamon for even fewer calories than a regular potato.

59. Cook white or brown rice without the butter that the box recipe calls for (it will taste the same).

HOMEMADE DESSERTS & SNACKS

60. Grease pans with nonfat cooking spray.

61. Use nonfat whipped toppings instead of icing.

62. Sprinkle nuts on top of items instead of mixing into batters.

63. Substitute 6 egg whites and 1 whole egg for every 3 eggs in your favorite recipes.

64. Use applesauce for some of the oil in your favorite recipes. Use 1/2 oil and 1/2 applesauce for best results.

65. Bake items with cocoa powder instead of chocolate.

66. Eat homemade fruit salad instead of apple pie.

67. Make milk shakes with nonfat yogurt, skim milk, ice, bananas and berries in a blender.

68. Eat pretzels instead of chips.

69. Watch out for fattier pretzels that contain cheese, butter and other ingredients.

70. Buy baked, not fried versions of chips and crackers.

71. Flavor air-popped popcorn with chili powder, herbs or salt substitute.

72. Eat fat-free angel food cake instead of pound cake.

73. Use fresh vegetables like celery, carrots, red peppers and broccoli as dip items.

74. Snack on bite size fruit like grapes or apple pieces instead of candies.

75. Freeze peeled banana chunks and washed grapes for a delicious alternative to ice cream.

76. Replace hot fudge with chocolate syrup on frozen yogurt.

77. Use wafers or sugar cones instead of waffle cones.

78. Top ice cream with sprinkles instead of chocolate candies.

79. Try fat-free sorbet or nonfat sherbet instead of ice cream.

80. Make ice pops at home by freezing juices in ice cube trays.

81. Dip fresh fruits like strawberries and pineapples in chocolate syrup to replace candy bars.

82. Replace chocolate-chip cookies with low-fat graham crackers and a little chocolate syrup.

83. Sugar-free hot cocoa will help satisfy a chocolate craving.

84. Purchase special desserts by the serving, not in large quantities.

AT THE MARKET

85. Be a label reader. Buy low-fat items whenever possible.

86. Look for cheeses such as ricotta, cottage, Swiss and mozzarella made from part-skim or skim milk.

87. Make your own iced tea and sweeten to taste with sugar substitutes.

88. Try apple butter instead of regular butter for breads & crackers.

89. Find reduced fat and nonfat versions of your favorite salad dressings.

90. Buy flavored seltzer waters instead of soda.

91. Buy water-based fruit not syrup packed.

92. Use unsweetened applesauce over the regular varieties.

93. Choose choice or extra-lean ground beef instead of prime.

94. Prepare ground meat dishes using turkey instead of beef.

95. Buy dehydrated soups made with baked (not fried) noodles.

96. Buy noodles made from semolina or durum wheat, not egg.

97. Compare the fat and calorie content on hotdog labels for leanness. Turkey or chicken franks are best.

98. Start with canned vegetarian baked beans and add your own pork, if desired.

99. Buy water packed tuna, not oil packed.

100. Stay away from purchasing packaged foods whenever possible. Buy fresh meats and produce.

101. Use whipped cottage cheese as a replacement for cream cheese.

chapter nine

What's a Food Group & Why You Care

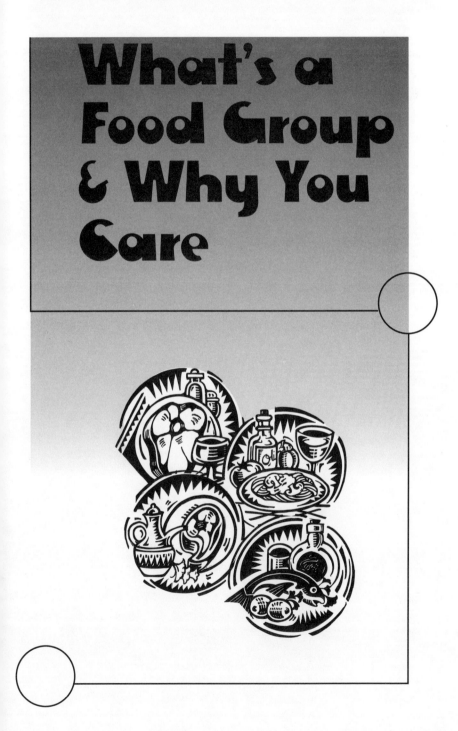

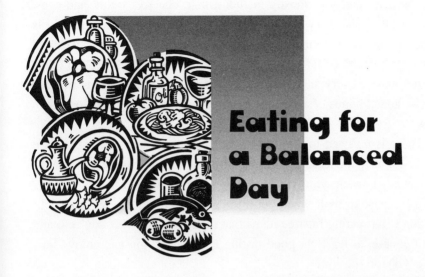

Eating for a Balanced Day

As I continually say throughout this book, I want you to learn to eat by category or food groups, rather than by counting calories. This takes away a lot of the potential for you to be constantly thinking about food throughout your day.

I'm sure your basic health classes have taught you that there are five basic food groups: Meat, dairy, fruit, vegetable, and starch & grain. Think of your meat group as your "Protein" group. This is the most important category to help your weight loss because you need to eat at least ten ounces of some sort of protein daily. I don't care if you eat more. I just don't want you to eat less than ten ounces. Protein can be in the form of chicken, turkey, seafood, veal or lean red meat. Protein also comes in other food categories such as dairy items like cheese and milk but I don't want to confuse the issue. We're going to make eating right as simple as possible.

Protein is not only important to help you lose weight, it's critical to your overall health. Every living cell, tissue, skin, bone, hair, blood, and muscle requires protein. It also helps the body build resistance to disease in the form of antibodies. Think of protein as the "high-test" fuel for your body.

The dairy category mostly includes milk, cheese, yogurt, and eggs. By controlling the dairy you eat, you can control a lot of fat since fat is found in most dairy items. If you're eating fat-free dairy items like skim milk, egg beaters, or fat-free yogurt, consider those to be protein items and not dairy. Dairy should be contained to about one serving per day with an added bonus of a glass of milk for your morning cereal or just to drink.

There is no need to give up flavor in the food you eat just to save calories. Fat-free cheese generally has the flavor and consistency of rubber bands! I swear, you will burn down your house before you can get fat-free cheese to melt when you're making a grilled cheese sandwich! So, don't start eating fat-free items that really taste bad. If you're going to eat cheese, at least eat good tasting cheese that you can enjoy - just don't 'OD' on the stuff!

The next food group is fruits. Fruit is tasty, light, generally has no fat content and usually contains a certain amount of acid that actually helps both digestion and fat burn. Most fruit is unlimited every day. Cantaloupe, oranges, apples, grapefruits, lemons, all fall into the unlimited category. High sugar fruits like watermelon, pineapple, plums, grapes, peaches, bananas and fruits like these should be limited to every-other day. That's because you don't want your body to have unnaturally high sugar levels because any sugar that's not burned off during the day, will ultimately turn into fat like it does with carbohydrates.

Fruits are delicious and nutritious, packed with vitamins and nutrients our bodies need. In fact, you should be eating at least two fruits every day. Eating any fruit is better than eating none, but some are better for you than others. Be sure to eat fresh fruit not canned. Processing fruit increases the sugar content, but lessens the fruit's nutritional value

Here are the ones I consider the "'Top 10 Fueling Fruits" that are exceptionally packed with good things for you:

Oranges top the list with high doses of vitamin C: an antioxidant that may fight or reduce bad cholesterol and cancer-causing diseases. Oranges also contain beta-carotene which is vitamin A as well as folic acid which helps prevent birth defects in the future and you can eat as many as you want every day!

Apricots are iron-packed and high in vitamins A and C, as well as potassium. Apricots are a great alternative for a "sweet tooth" because they will stop the body's sugar cravings so, give this one a try.

Tomatoes are actually a fruit even though we may think of them as a vegetable. They are filled with vitamins A and C as well as lycopene which is a substance that may help combat prostate cancer.

Cantaloupe is also one of your unlimited fruits that is full of potassium which helps regulate the heart. You should eat cantaloupe to help restore some of the potassium you will lose if you're exercising or playing hard. This is also a natural energy enhancer that contains vitamin A - a vitamin that is known to improve heart and muscle function.

Bananas are a fabulous source of minerals, vitamins, and potassium. Easy to digest, bananas are a fast source of energy and even help eliminate leg cramps.

Mangoes are loaded with vitamin C and beta-carotene. Both of which boost the immune system.

Grapefruit is a good source of beta-carotene and vitamin C. Red or pink should be chosen if you are looking for the most nutrition and sweetest flavor.

Strawberries and Blueberries provide you with more fiber than two slices of whole wheat bread and are high in vitamin C.

Kiwi is also a good source of vitamin C and is high in potassium. Sweet and delicious, two large kiwis contain more fiber than a cup of bran!

Depending on where you live, eating fruit every day can be hard, especially in the winter months.

If you're not a big fruit eater, you might try adding it to yogurt or a protein shake. Eating whole fruit is much more filling and nutritious than juicing it and making it into a drink so try to eat fruits fresh and in their natural form whenever you can. It's not unusual for most of the 'good stuff' like vitamins and minerals to be found in the pulp or skins which can be lost in juicing. And, when I tell you about the health benefits of some of these items, like cancer-fighter or antioxidant, it's not to scare you. The more you know about food now, the more motivated you will be to continue to eat right as you get older. Don't be afraid of facts and information. You'll be amazed at how handy it is to be smart!

I sort of lump fruits & vegetables into the same category. If you're not a big steamed vegetable fan, have a salad. That will at least boost your body with an excellent form of beta-carotene and fiber.

Now we come to starches & grains OR your "carbohydrate category." I know, first hand, that this one is tough. I personally could live on breads and pasta, but I think you'll better understand why this is a problem when you realize that it takes 15 minutes of jogging for your body to eliminate 1 slice of low-calorie bread. Think about it. If you have a bowl of cereal for breakfast, a sub-sandwich for lunch and spaghetti for dinner, you'll be jogging for the next week to burn off the sugar that those starch/carbohydrates produced in just one day!

Just for the record, the carbohydrate category (carbs for those "in-the-know!") contains all of your rice, bread, pasta, potato, corn, cereal, crackers, cookies and starchy items. For this category, you can have two servings every day. If you choose to eat cereal for breakfast and a sandwich for lunch, then try to stay away from any bread, rice or pasta at dinnertime.

Weight loss is about making choices. If you know that you may only eat 2 carb items each day, you need to select which meals are better or most likely to include carbs. Personally, I love carbohydrates but I try to make sure that I make my carbs really count. Once again, it's what I call "worth it" foods. I rarely eat sandwiches anymore because I'd rather eat a really great dinner roll, or a side of pasta rather than 'waste' my favorite two allowable servings each day on sandwich bread. Obviously, this philosophy only works if you are in a position to eat something other than a sandwich at lunchtime.

Finding good food alternatives that satisfy your hunger and taste good isn't difficult. It just takes a little information and a little practice. For example, breakfast doesn't have to mean cereal. You can have fruit, eggs, breakfast meats, a hamburger patty, Jell-O, cottage cheese, or yogurt to start your day.

Even though I really want you to start making exercise a regular part of your life, the more you can learn to stay away from starch items, the faster, easier and more effective your weight loss effort will be.

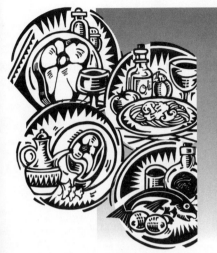

What are Proteins, Carbohydrates and Fats?

I think it's always easier to make changes or eat certain things when you understand the reason or benefit behind what you're doing. When you learn how your body benefits from these three food groups, it will make it a lot easier for you to eat them in the balance that will do your body the most good.

PROTEIN

This is the most important food group of all. For the most part, protein is found in your meat food group. It's in foods like beef, veal, fish, poultry, cheese, eggs and tofu. I'd like you to choose foods from the lean meat category over the higher fat meats as often as possible so you can keep the fat and calories that you're eating nice and low.

Here's a few protein pointers: Even though it tastes really good, you need to try not to eat the skin of the meat or poultry because it's full of fat. I also want you to eat only fresh meats from the butcher shop whenever possible and not the processed luncheon meat found in plastic wrap in the deli case. If the meat is not processed, the fat content should be less than 30% which is completely acceptable and very good for you.

The reason it is so important to eat at least ten ounces of protein every day is because protein plays a very important role in your body. Protein is a part of every living cell and makes up tissue, skin, bone, hair, blood and muscle. If you don't eat enough protein, cells can't function properly or be repaired. Protein also plays a significant role in the following body processes:

- Building new body tissue.
- Repairing worn-out tissue.
- Providing a source of energy and heat for the body.
- Contributing to the composition of the body's fluids.
- Transporting substances through the blood stream.
- Helps with building resistance to disease in the formation of antibodies.

Amino acids are the building blocks of protein. Some non-essential amino acids are produced by the body, but essential amino acids must be supplied to you by the food you eat. Just to be sure your diet is chock-full of all twenty-two necessary amino acids (which you are never going to personally calculate!), eat a variety of foods that are full of protein every day.

CARBOHYDRATES & STARCHES

These are the foods you probably eat the most and need to cut down on the most! Carbohydrates are found in breads, grains, pasta, crackers, sugars, milk, as well as some fruits and vegetables. You don't need to even think about the carbs that can be found in fruits & vegetables. Those are complex-carbs which are really good for you, and don't have the same impact on your body as starch-type carbohydrates such as pasta, bread and crackers. Carbohydrates also provide the body with a good source of fiber which it needs.

Although the body likes carbs best as as source of energy, it will turn to other sources of energy if it doesn't have enough carbs to pull from. Protein is the usual alternate source for energy, and that's why I want you to eat lots of protein.

Here's a little body chemistry lesson: After you eat a potato (which is a starch-carb), your body breaks the potato down in the digestive process. The starch of the potato is turned into glucose which is a form of sugar. Glucose is needed by all living cells and provides the body with the "fuel" it needs to operate smoothly.

If a person is inactive or doesn't exercise very much, they need to eat fewer carbohydrates (no more than two servings daily) because the unused glucose or sugar that the carbs create will ultimately turn to fat in the body. If you exercise regularly, this is not a big problem and you can eat an additional carbohydrate serving. If you exercise very little or not at all and continue to eat a lot of carbs, this is what happens: Most of the carbs you have eaten have no way to get burned off because of your inactivity. All the carbs will turn into sugar. A small portion of the sugar will be used to give your body energy, the leftover sugar will ultimately turn into fat. When the sugar your body makes is greater than the sugar your body uses, your body then becomes a fat manufacturing machine! Isn't that GROSS?

FATS

Fats are found in margarine, butter, oils, nuts, salad dressings, cream, and items like these. Most of these contain what I call "bad fat." "Good fats" are found in meats, poultry and fish but the fat content there should not concern you because they are 'good.' Good fats are the essential fats that your body needs. Although it is important to limit your intake of fat, a small amount should be included in your daily diet because fat serves an important role in many body functions such as:

• Providing the body with energy.
• Carrying vitamins A, D, E, and K throughout the body.
• Helping vitamins be absorbed.
• Helping form cells in the body.
• Providing padding which protects internal organs from
  damage.
• Helping maintain skin tissue.

Remember, your body needs fat. If you attempt to be fat-free, you will die! Just be sure that you are eating good fats like essential fatty acids found in proteins and keep the bad fats found in processed foods to a minimum. Eating fresh stuff tastes so much better and is much better for you. Stay away from anything processed whenever you can. Learn to read product labels so you know what's in the food you eat. If the ingredients list a bunch of words you've never heard of or can't pronounce, don't eat it!

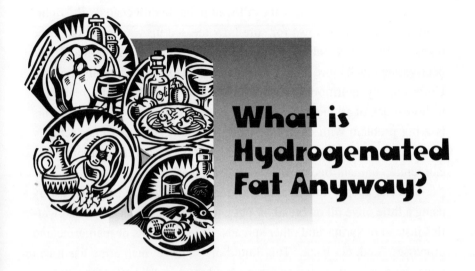

What is Hydrogenated Fat Anyway?

As a rule of thumb, try not to eat anything if you don't know what it is! A lot of fast food and higher fat snack items contain hydrogenated oils. These oils are made by adding hydrogen to corn, soybean or other liquid oils to make them more solid and stable and to provide food manufacturers with a cheaper oil for their products. Just so you understand the impact this kind of oil can have on you, Dr. Walter Willet, a Harvard researcher, estimated that 30,000 of the deaths each year from heart disease could be prevented if we would cut back or eliminate the use of hydrogenated fats in our diets. Makes you wonder how an ingredient like this can still be legal to use, doesn't it?

Besides margarine, manufacturers use hydrogenated oils in pre-packaged pudding to give it a creamy consistency. Yummmmy! Hydrogenated oils are also used in crackers, cookies, potato chips and many other foods so they can sit on a grocery store shelf longer. Hydrogenated oils are often used for deep-frying in fast food restaurants because they are less likely to turn rancid or spoil.

How Much Of These Oils Can We Eat?

I bet, right about now, you can't wait to eat hydrogenated oils, right? Well, no one really knows for sure how messed up your body could be thanks to these oils, but we do know that in recent years, Americans have been eating much more manufactured fats than experts originally thought. Unfortunately, nutrition labels are misleading since they don't really tell us how much of all the different kinds of fat are in the foods we eat. This is a big problem with consumer label programs...one that may actually cause food processors to use more bad fats over saturated fat since fats can remain unidentified on the label. Isn't that scary?

You can keep hydrogenated and trans-fats as low as possible just by using a little olive oil on bread, or put jam or honey on pancakes and waffles instead of syrups and other spreads. If you eat lots of margarine and processed food, cut back. Tub, liquid or 'squeeze' margarine has much lower fat content than the stick-type, but butter is still better for you than anything else. When cooking or baking, use non-stick sprays, olive oil or applesauce instead of margarine or butter. Herb mixtures or lemon juice give a lot of extra flavor to steamed vegetables and you won't miss the butter here either.

The bottom line is to be aware of the fat content in everything you eat. Keep fats to 30% of the calorie count per serving if it's listed on the package, and you'll automatically consume fewer hidden fats too.

chapter ten

You've Got Options

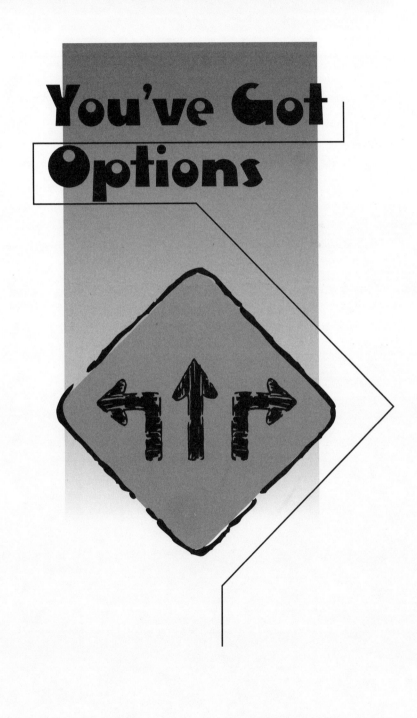

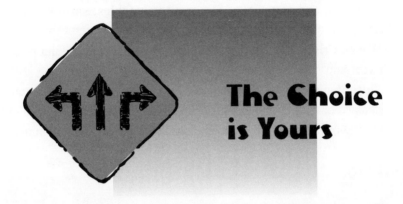

The Choice is Yours

I know you've figured out by now that you are in control of what you eat. If you're at home, your options may be a little easier to control. If you're eating out, most restaurants usually offer meals for health-conscious diners. To help you make better decisions, I'm giving you some lighter options and high-fat pitfalls offered by the American Heart Association and Center for Science in the Public Interest.

"Best" choices have less than 30 grams of fat. "Worst" have up to 100 grams. POINT OF INFORMATION: There are 9 calories to every fat gram. You'll learn more about this in the "Learn to Calculate Fats" section of this book.

FAST FOOD

Best: Grilled chicken sandwich, roast beef sandwich, single hamburger or salad with light vinaigrette dressing.

Worst: Baconburger, double cheeseburger, french fries, onion rings and chicken wings.

Tips: Order sandwiches without mayo or 'special sauces.' Avoid deep-fried items like fish filets and chicken nuggets.

CHINESE

Best: Hot-and-sour soup. Stir-fried vegetables, shrimp w/garlic sauce, Szechwan shrimp, wonton soup.
Worst: Crispy chicken or duck, kung pao chicken, moo shu pork & sweet-and-sour anything!
Tips: Share a stir-fry with steamed rice not fried. Ask for vegetables steamed or stirred with less oil. Have moo shu vegetables or chicken instead of pork. Avoid breaded dishes and items that contain nuts.

ITALIAN

Best: Pasta with red or white clam sauce, spaghetti with marinara or tomato w/meat sauce.
Worst: Anything "parmigiana," fettuccini alfredo, fried calamari, lasagna.
Tips: Stick with plain bread not garlic bread and try to eat pasta on the side of a dish containing chicken, beef or seafood rather than an entree.

Even pizza is not terrible if you don't pile it high with pepperoni and cheese. Salads can become fatty if you include lots of cheese and processed meat then soak it in an oily salad dressing.

SANDWICHES

Best: Ham & swiss, roast beef, turkey.
Worst: Tuna salad, reuben, submarine.
Tips: Use mustard or catsup instead of mayo and hold the cheese.

MEXICAN

Best: Bean burrito (no cheese), chicken or beef fajitas.
Worst: Beef chimichanga, chile relleño, quesadilla.
Tips: Choose soft tortillas with fresh salsa. Stay away from guacamole.

Black beans are much better than refried beans. You can also have grilled shrimp, fish or chicken.

SEAFOOD

Best: Broiled bass, halibut, snapper, scallops, steamed crab or lobster.
Worst: Fried anything! Blackened catfish.
Tips: Have fish broiled, baked, grilled or steamed. Do not pan fry or sauté. Use lemon instead of tartar sauce and avoid butter.

Be sensible when selecting your food. If you think it may be high in fat, then it probably is. Just think before you eat and you won't go wrong.

HELPFUL TIP:

If you want to lose weight fast and easy, a simple-to-remember rule of thumb is to limit what you eat if it contains any of the following:

• Bubbles (like soda)
• Butter & oils
• Processed, fried & frozen food
• Salt & soy sauce
• Rolls & muffins
• Whole milk & cream
• Caffeine & chocolate

It is a lot easier to make good food choices when you know more about food. Most people think we want to eat our favorite foods. The fact is, the foods we eat BECOME our favorites because that's what we get used to. You can change your tastebuds and enjoy food that's good for you when you know more about what you eat and what you should avoid.

Like their parents, most kids are victims of habit, go with the flow and eat on the run. That's why you tend to eat the same basic "fast food" things most of the time. I want to tell you a little bit more about the 10 most popular foods American's eat and why it might be a really good idea for you to consider changing a few of your "habits".

What you decide to eat is certainly your business. But, at least do it 'heads-up'. Do you have to eliminate the items on this list forever? No... but, the less you eat of them, the healthier and leaner you will be. That's all. Getting in shape and being healthy is a choice not a requirement. God only gave you one body and you have to live with it for a very long time. Cancer, diabetes and heart disease don't just happen. YOU "grow them" by feeding and encouraging their growth and development eating cancer-causing chemicals, man-made fats and unnatural sugars that are hidden in your "favorite foods".

AMERICA'S FAVORITES

1, 2 & 3: Hamburgers, Hot Dogs & Chicken Nuggets

• All of these foods are put in the "high risk" food category by the government because of the poor heath standards they are manufactured under.

• It takes a lot of time to process meat in burger, dog or nugget form. That's why processed meats like these have high bacteria counts. Putrefaction or rotting of the meat also takes place during the manu facturing process which needs to be treated with chemicals and drugs.

• As the meat begins to decompose, it turns green. Because green meat would not be too appetizing in the store, meat producers dye it with red chemicals so it appears fresh. Unless marked otherwise, ground hamburger and hot dogs will always contain red dyes.

• Hamburgers, hotdogs and chicken nuggets are made with the unusable, worst leftovers of the slaughterhouse...much of which comes right off the floor. Any meat "part" that cannot be sold on its own like steaks and chops is ground up and used. This includes hooves, bone, snout, ears, beak, feet and other animal parts.

• Because all parts of hamburger, hotdogs or processed chicken come from an animal, "pure beef", "100% turkey" or "all chicken" can be used on the label.

• Most of these three food items contain the flavor enhancer, "MSG" (monosodium glutamate) which causes headaches and allergic reactions. MSG is a chemical used to fatten up laboratory animals and will ultimately make you fat when you eat it yourself. Even though you are not eating it intentionally, you are still eating MSG when it is contained in the food you choose to eat.

- The beef industry is the largest user of antibiotics in the world. Antibiotics are used to fight the dangerous bacteria that is growing in the meat during the time the dead animal is made into hamburger, hotdogs or chicken nuggets. The bad part about the use of antibiotics for this purpose is that it has caused many Americans to build up a tolerance for antibiotics so when they need them for other health reasons, they no longer work. Their body becomes immune to the effects of germ-fighting drugs.

- Ground beef is more likely to harbor life-threatening E-coli bacteria than any other food.

- Hamburgers are the single biggest food item that inflicts the most damage on the American diet....Billions served....billions spent on doctor visits and hospital bills!

- The hormones fed to cattle can make you fat by eating the meat from that animal.

- A Cheeseburger contains more than 100% of your TOTAL daily recommended fat intake!

- Burger King's Double Whopper with cheese has 1150 calories and 76 grams of fat with 33 of them saturated, plus a whopping 1,530 mg. of sodium!

- Burger condiments like pickle, lettuce, tomato, etc. are all treated with cancer- causing chemical sulfites that are used so the lettuce and other vegetable items stay fresh and don't turn brown.

- Most burgers contain 1090 mg of sodium! (45% of daily recommended Daily Value) and can cause your body to store water which will make you puffy and uncomfortable.

- Both turkey and beef hotdogs, have nitrites which are thought to cause stomach cancer, leukemia, brain tumors, and bladder cancer.

- Meat processors use fillers and non-meat binders to hold hot dog meat together. These binders may be cereal, non-fat dry milk, or soy which adds more carbohydrates and processed ingredients when you think you're just eating meat.

- Synthetic collagen casings with no nutritional value are used to form and shape hot dogs.

- Up to 40% of a hot dog and 50% of chicken nuggets are made up of

- When the buns for hotdogs and hamburgers are baked, or chicken nuggets are deep fried, they release a powerful toxin called acrylimides which is a known cancer agent that causes nerve damage and cancer.

- Chicken nuggets are heavily breaded so they look like bigger pieces of chicken which adds a lot of carbohydrates to what you think is just protein.

- Chicken nuggets contain phosphates which make the body have more acid. A high acid content in the body makes it almost impossible for you to burn fat properly. You will store fat and not lose weight.

- Some chicken nuggets (McDonalds) contain aluminum which is toxic to the brain and poisons the metabolism. Anytime your metabolism slows down, weight loss becomes much more difficult.

- Any item deep fried is usually cooked in oxidized oil that is re-used for weeks at a time! Saturated fats that are probably not told to you on the label.

4. French Fries:

- French fries are very toxic and harmful to your body.

- In order to make French fries, they must be cooked at high temperatures in hot oils which cause the chemical, acrylimide to be released. Remember, acrylimides are a known cancer-causing agent that also causes nerve damage.

- Potatoes are grown in the ground. In order to keep bugs away from the vegetables, farmers spray pesticides which are poisons that keep the bugs out. Unfortunately, potatoes and many other vegetables soak up a lot of the nutrients from the soil and when pesticides are on that soil, the potatoes soak that up too. In fact, potatoes have a high er absorption level than almost any other food product.

- Fries are cooked in oxidized oil that is re-used for weeks at a time.

- Potatoes have a very high glycemic index meaning it turns to sugar very quickly in your body. Eating a baked potato (or French fries of about the same amount) has the same sugar-punch to your body as if you ate a large piece of chocolate cake! Even though the potato may not contain fat directly, the unused sugar created from the chemistry of the potato will ultimately turn to fat in your body.

5. Oreo Cookies:
THE NUMBER ONE COOKIE IN AMERICA (6 cookies is a serving size)

- Oreos are mostly made up of 23 grams of straight-line sugar.

- Chocolate is the LAST ingredient listed which means chocolate is the least of the ingredients used in each Oreo cookie.

- 370 empty calories with almost no nutritional benefits - you could eat 2 whole chicken breasts for the same amount of calories in a serving of Oreos!

- 6 cookies have 12 grams of fat, 2.5 grams of saturated fat and 40 carbs - more than 50% of your daily carbohydrate allowance in only 6 cookies.

- After you eat Oreo cookies, your body will crave more sugar within 3 hours!

- "Natural flavors" are not real flavors at all and they are certainly NOT natural. They are manufactured chemicals to make Oreos taste like great chocolate cookies. Highly processed foods use chemicals which they call "flavor enhancers" that make food taste better. Unfortunately, "flavor enhancers" are actually cancer-causing chemicals with no natural flavors of their own can cause cancer and other physical ailments.

- The Nabisco Company refused to tell us how many transfats, which are dangerous hidden fats, are in Oreo cookies - Nabisco termed that information as 'classified'! Why shouldn't we know what we are eating? Is it THAT dangerous!?

- Oreo cookies have a high sugar content. Sugar causes facial wrinkles and dimpling of legs, thighs and buttocks.

6. Pizza:

- Most commercial pizzas are made exclusively of 5 genetically modified foods and do not contain real ingredients like fresh tomato and cheese:

  - Cheese "food" (Contains only 10% cheese - it cannot even be called   real cheese)

  - Enriched white flour which has been bleached of natural vitamins and minerals BUT has been "enriched" by adding back a very little amount of synthetic or 'fake' vitamins in its place.

- Tomato sauce made from tomato-like substances, not fresh tomatoes, that produce their own pesticides, IN YOU!

- Wheat in the pizza crust is genetically modified and not natural.

- Contains cottonseed oil. Cotton is not a "food" so it can be sprayed with anything farmers want to keep bugs and bacteria away. Farmers have a lot more limits to what they can spray on food items they are growing. The seed from the cotton carries most of the poison of the cotton plant. The USDA and the FDA do not cooperate with each other in making sure this is safe to eat. It is not. Plus, it is highly hydrogenated which means the fat in cottonseed oil is man-made, dense and dangerous to your health.

- Pizza is baked at such a high temperature, the crust will form cancer-causing acrylimides.

- Pepperoni & sausage toppings are "high risk" processed meats which add lots of nitrites, chemicals, preservatives, and saturated fats to your food.

7. Soda:

- The active ingredient in Coke is phosphoric acid. On the Ph scale, it has so much acid that it can dissolve a nail in about 4 days!

- High acid content in the body makes it very difficult to lose weight.

- Soda will drain the calcium out of your bones which promotes osteo porosis - a disease that makes bones brittle and break easily.

- There are 10-12 teaspoons of empty-calorie sugar in one can of soda.

- Diet sodas with artificial sweeteners will make you have more sugar cravings because sweeteners are "sweeter" than sugar.

- Colorings used in sodas are cancer-causing and unnatural.

- Soda is called "liquid candy" because of the high sugar content. It's like drinking a candy bar!

- High fructose corn syrup is a major ingredient in soda and:

  - Damages proteins in your body.

  - Be stored in the body as fat.

  - Is made from corn, which is a modified food that produces its own pesticides.

8. Ice cream:

- High in fat content. 1 serving (usually 4 ounces which is smaller than most ice cream stores serve) can provide as much as 50% of your recommended fat for the day.

- High in carbohydrates. 1 serving is almost 40% of your total recommended carb intake for the day.

- High in sugar which promotes sugar cravings and causes skin to wrinkle and dimple.

- Full of hydrogenated and transfats which are unnatural and:
  - elevate cholesterol and bad fat levels
  - clog arteries
  - create free radicals (which may cause cancer)

- Hormones put into cows to make them produce more milk will slow your metabolism, and can cause breast and ovarian tumors, cysts and cancer later in life.

9. Donuts:

- The average donut contains approximately 300 calories.

- 1 donut provides more than 50% of your recommended daily carbohydrate intake.

- Donuts are high in salt content which will cause you to store water in your body. You will see the extra water as swollen hands & feet.

- Donuts are deep fried in oxidized oil that is re-used for weeks at a time!

- Dunkin Donuts changes the oil every 300 dozen donuts!

- Oils at high temperatures developed rancidity and free radicals which can:

  - Poison and slow your metabolism

  - Seriously threaten your health.

  - Donuts have a high sugar content which promotes sugar cravings and ages skin.

10. Potato Chips: America's #1 snack food

Americans today eat more potato chips than any other people in the world. As a world food, potatoes are the second most eaten food. Rice is #1.

- It takes 4 pounds of potatoes to make 1 pound of potato chips.

- Chips have a lot of calories for their small size. A small 2 oz. bag has over 300 calories!

- Potato chips are deep fried in oxidized oil that is re-used for weeks at a time.

- Chips are deep fried at high temperatures which cause the chemical, acrylimide to be released.

- When you eat 1 single serving bag of potato chips you may be eating up to 500 times more acrylamide than the maximum level allowed in drinking water.

- A single potato chip could contain as much acrylamide as the government allows for an 8-ounce glass of drinking water!

- Chips are high in hidden saturated fats.

- Chips have a high sodium/salt content that makes your body store water.

"HEALTHY CHIPS" LIKE BAKED LAYS OR THOSE CONTAINING OLESTRA CAN BE MORE DANGEROUS TO YOUR HEALTH THAN REGULAR CHIPS.

- Baked Lays have almost as many calories as original Lays. They are a highly processed mixture of dehydrated potato and food starch pressed into a chip shape and are full of cancer-causing chemicals.

- Olean/Olestra potato chips. Can cause "anal oil leakage" or a variety of stomach problems, as reported on the bag.

- Fake fats like Olean or Olestra block fat absorption in the body which doesn't let your body absorb valuable nutrients contained in the healthy foods you eat.

- When you eat something that encourages your body to change the way it processes the food you eat, you can't control what that change effects. Even though you may only want to stop fat from being absorbed in your body, fake fats like these also stops your body from properly absorbing valuable nutrients that protect your body from heart disease, cancer and other diseases.

"How does the government let this happen?" you might ask. "Why are these foods available to us if they are so bad?" Simple. Food is big business. Zillions of dollars are made in America off people who eat in fast food restaurants or buy "junk" food.

It is also important for you to realize that it's not your fault if you tend to eat a lot of the items that are on this list. You have been the target of people selling these kinds of foods from the time you were a little baby. Back in the 1950's, when fast food like McDonald's started, people didn't know how harmful it really was. Moms & dads thought they were doing something fun and easy when they took you to a fast food restaurant. Never did America think that they would pay a gigantic price for convenience. Unfortunately, it doesn't stop there. Portion sizes keep getting bigger too. Because food manufacturers know that you would feel like a pig if you ate two hamburgers or an extra order of French fries, they simply made the portion size twice as big and created "Value Meals". What a trick! It let America eat more without the guilt.

My goal is to make you think about what you eat at the earliest age possible and question anything that does not appear to make sense to you. If you do that, you'll not only be a better shopper when you get older, you will also be a healthier one. Look at the labels for anything you eat and try to eat foods that don't come in boxes, cans or plastic wraps. Anything that comes in some sort of package usually means that it has some kind of chemical in it that will make the food stay fresh for a long time. When you think about it, does it really make sense that a cookie or cake can stay "fresh" for over a year as long as it remains packaged? How can that be? The cakes and cookies your mom or grandma make can't stay fresh for more than about a week. Store-bought sweets aren't magical, they're just full of chemicals that can hurt you. So, when in doubt, don't eat 'em!

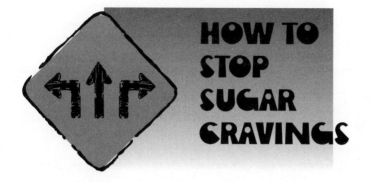

HOW TO STOP SUGAR CRAVINGS

It is scary to think that the average American eats 147 pounds of sugar every year! Kids included! And, it can be addicting! Your body is one big chemical machine. When you eat sugar, you are eating empty calories that have none of the nutrients, minerals and vitamins your body needs to burn itself up. In order for sugar to get used in the body, it steals nutrients from other sources and messes up your body's energy production, fat metabolism, heat production, and general activity. It also affects your brain chemistry by sending temporary signals to your brain that says you "feel good". Once that signal wears off, your body craves more sugar so it can "feel good" again.

Eating sweets is not the only way to increase sugar levels in the body either. Insulin is the master hormone in your body. Sugars and starches produce insulin. When your body makes too much insulin, it converts sugar & starch into fat instead of burning fat as fuel. Starchy carbohydrates like rice, bread, potatoes and pasta all make sugar (or glucose) that causes your body to crave more. Most people find they are hungry for more food within three hours of having desserts or starchy carbs like cereal or bagels. The best way to eliminate sugar cravings is to eliminate the foods that make your body want more sugar.

179

INSULIN AFFECTS EVERYTHING

If you find you have sugar cravings a lot of the time, you probably have an insulin imbalance. That means your 'master hormone' is overloaded and not working as it should. When this happens:

- You have trouble losing weight
- Too much insulin makes you hungrier.
- An insulin imbalance will cause your body to store and keep unwanted fat.
- Insulin is created by eating sugars OR starches - both types of foods can be just as big a problem for your body.
- You do NOT need to eat sweets in order to have insulin problems.
- Insulin problems can lead to juvenile and adult diabetes.

You might think that a cookie or soda isn't such a big deal. But, it really is if cookies and sodas are a regular part of your daily diet. These kinds of sugary foods impact your body more than you can imagine. We already have sugar in our bodies. The body produces it all by itself. When we add more, it just causes problems.

Let me give you an example of what sugar can do to an 14 year old. The average 14 year old has a normal sugar level in their blood stream equal to 5 grams of sugar. That is what a healthy 14 year old system should have. That sugar level can be created by the 14 year olds own body and does not need him or her to consume any more sugar in order for their body to have just the right amount that it needs. But, if that 14 year old drinks 1 soda, they have now added as much as 40 grams of sugar to their blood system - 6-8 times more than what their body wanted or needed. So, if you eat a sugar frosted cereal for breakfast, a soda for lunch, candy bar in the afternoon and a soda plus dessert at dinner, you will have eaten, in one day, the blood sugar level necessary to keep 20 or more 14-year olds alive!

If you have behavior problems, attention deficits (ADD/ADHD), have a hard time focusing on what the teacher says in class, or can't remember things very well, you are probably eating too much sugar. Sugar or too much insulin in your body can affect you in these kinds of ways. Changing the way you eat will also affect how you feel and even the way you think.

Let me give you another example. A scientific team did a study with school kids that gave the kids a specific exam in the morning and the exact same exam in the afternoon. Since the kids already knew what would be on the afternoon test, it was expected that they would score better on the afternoon exam. Each child was given a healthy, high protein breakfast, then they were tested. The afternoon exam came shortly after the kids had eaten a Twinkie and soda with their lunch. Even though the kids took the same exam twice and knew the test questions beforehand, their test scores dropped 16-20% LOWER than their morning scores. The only difference between the morning and afternoon tests was the lunchtime sugar the children ate.

So, now what do you do? By eating a lot of fruits, vegetables and protein, and staying away from starchy carbohydrates like bread and pasta as much as you can, you will quickly keep your body's insulin levels more even. When your insulin level stops jumping up and down, your cravings for sugar will go away too.

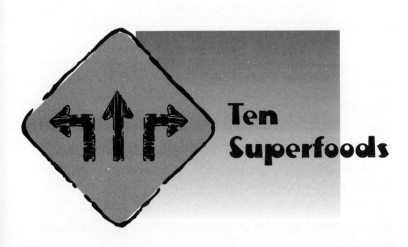

Ten Superfoods

When you're young, the thought of eating foods that will help prevent diseases seems pretty unnecessary. But, not all foods are created equal. Some are really 'super' and help keep your body stronger and healthier. The ones that I've listed are nutritional powerhouses, or chocked-full of disease preventers, or both. All are low in fat and calories. They are easily available and intensely good for you.

I know some of these are going to seem kinda yucky to you and you may have never even thought about eating them before now, but, give them a shot. And, don't be surprised if you even start to like some of them! OH, NOOOOOO!

1. **Broccoli** contains at least 4 substances that have anti-cancer properties and other elements in this green giant to help keep cholesterol levels steady and protect your heart. Stop yawning! I'm really serious about all of this! Ounce for ounce, broccoli contains as much calcium as milk.

2. **Yogurt** has been associated with preventing yeast infections, strengthening the immune system, balancing intestinal bacteria (nice thought) if you happen to be taking any

antibiotics and   even preventing cancer. It contains more calcium than milk and aids the digestion of lactose found in milk products.

3. **Wheat germ and bran** are considered the anti-cancer fibers since they reduce the risk of colon and breast cancers more effectively than oat or corn bran. Eating wheat germ or bran in cereal form provides you with a higher concentration of fiber, and less carbohydrate bulk.

4. **Papaya and papaya juice** contain enzymes that help you digest meat and milk proteins. Studies have shown that papaya is effective against ulcers and is also an excellent source of potassium and fiber.

5. **Strawberries** are high in fruit fiber, which reduces cholesterol levels, risk of hypertension (stress) and may prevent colon cancer. One half cup of strawberries actually provides more fiber than a slice of whole wheat bread.

6. **Tofu** contains a slew of healthful compounds. Some stimulate the immune system, and others may prevent several types of cancer and tumor growths. Tofu is an excellent source of protein with far fewer calories and fat grams than beef.

KEEP GOING...You're learning something!

7. **Onion and garlic** both lower high blood pressure, reduce dangerous blood clotting and lower bad cholesterol levels. Onions are considered to inhibit tumor formation and lessen bronchial asthma. Garlic contains an antibiotic and decongestant compound and has been shown to boost the immune system.

8. **Sweet potatoes** may help prevent cancer and reduce the plaque build-up that clogs arteries. One average-size sweet potato gives young ladies more than three times a female's daily requirement for vitamin A, and is also a good source of fiber, potassium, iron, and vitamins C and B6. Tasty without a lot of trimmings, sweet potato is a great carbohydrate.

9. **Tuna,** America's favorite fish, is rich in essential fatty acids which lowers cholesterol, reduces blood pressure, protects against strokes and alleviates migraines. Best eaten fresh or water-packed.

10. **Parsley** is the overlooked garnish laden with minerals so eat it when you get some on your plate! It's full of iron, copper, magnesium and boron which help reduce plaque in the arteries and fights mid-day 'snoozies' which can hit boron-deficient folks.

You made it! Don't be afraid to try stuff you haven't eaten before. You won't know how much you like things you've never tried, and, when they're also good for you, it's a bonus!

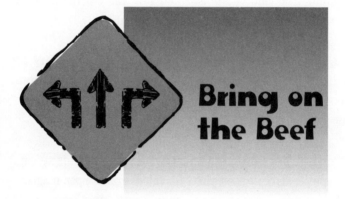

Bring on the Beef

A lot of people think eating beef isn't good for them and they should stick to eating fish or chicken. That's not correct. Beef has had good and bad publicity over the years, but the fact is, when it comes to mass-produced meats like beef, chicken or turkey, they all contain the same kinds of hormones and chemicals, therefore it doesn't make a lot of difference which one you choose.

If you're tired of chicken and turkey, don't be afraid to add meat to your menu. If you pick the leanest cuts and don't eat the fat around the edges, beef can be as light and lean as skinless chicken.

Just to show you how good beef can be for you, the fat gram numbers I'm showing here are for a 7 ounce piece of meat which is the serving size you'll get in most restaurants. Choose any of the items listed.

I didn't include ground beef or hamburger in my list because even extra-lean ground beef still has about 50% fat without adding mayonnaise or cheese. Stick with butcher cut meats like steaks and roasts.

BEEF - extra lean "select" grade, trimmed of fat - 7 oz. broiled

	fat grams
Eye of round	7.0
Top round	8.0
Top sirloin	11.2
Round tip	11.8
Top loin	13.8
Tenderloin	17.6

CHICKEN - fryer, 7 oz. roasted

Breast without skin	7.2
Drumstick without skin	11.4
Breast with skin	15.6
Thigh without skin	21.8
Drumstick with skin	22.4
Thigh with skin	31.8
Wing with skin	70.8

PORK - trimmed of fat, 7 oz. roasted

Tenderloin	9.6
Ham with bone	11.0
Chop-top loin	14.4

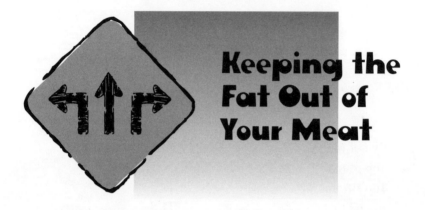

Keeping the Fat Out of Your Meat

If you're into cooking, you can make a nice piece of meat taste great and still keep the fat down with these cooking tips:

- Trim visible fat.

- Marinate in lime juice, and vinegar or nonfat yogurt for at least 2 hours.

- Cook meat quickly and on high heat.

- To broil or grill, cut the meat across the grain into 1/4-1/2" thick slices. Rub with herbs or brush with sauce regularly.

- When stir-frying, cook meat rapidly then remove. Cook vegetables separately so they don't soak up the fat from the meat. Add meat back after vegetables are cooked.

- Cook in non-stick pan or use vegetable spray for coating.

If you aren't good at cooking, share these tips with mom and encourage her to make foods lighter and healthier for you. I've found that all family members usually share bad habits, so your family might possibly benefit from a little guidance from you.

Don't be afraid to speak up. After all, you're becoming an expert on the subject of healthy eating!

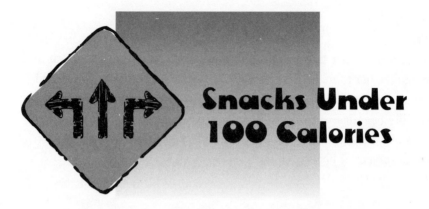

Snacks Under 100 Calories

It isn't realistic to think that you won't snack anymore. Snacking's a part of life and you're not going to stop. You also have a lot of snack options that won't put extra pounds on you. My suggestion is to keep snacks in the 200 calories-per-day range, so here are a few things you can eat that are still under 100 calories and very low in fat:

		Calories
Applesauce	1/2 cup	53
Apricots (fresh)	3	51
Blueberries	1 cup	80
Brownie (fat-free)	1	100
Cantaloupe	2 cups	75
String Cheese	1 oz.	80
Cottage Cheese	1/2 cup	80
Animal Crackers	7	60
Ritz Bitz Crackers	22	70
Saltine Crackers	6	75
Townhouse Crackers	5	80
Frozen Yogurt Fruit Bar	1	50
Fudgesicle (fat-free)	1	30

		Calories
Gum Drops	6	50
Hershey's Kisses	2	49
Vanilla Ice Milk	1/2 cup	90
Jell-O (sugar-free)	1 cup	20
Mini Marshmallows	10	25
Popcorn (air-popped)	3 cups	75
Popsicles (sugar-free)	3	75
Pretzel	1 large	55
Raisins	2 Tbs.	54
Rice Cakes	2	70
Rye Krisp	2	70
Thin Mints	2	84
Watermelon	1 cup	50
Entenmanns' fat-free cakes	1 oz.	90
Chocolate Covered Cherries	3	90
Gummy Bears	4	20
Nilla Wafer Cookies	4	90
Cheese Nips	13	70
Goldfish Crackers	30	90
Hard-Boiled Egg	1	79
Fruit Cocktail (canned in juice)	1/2 cup	56
Sorbet (fruit flavors)	1/2 cup	100
Weight Watchers Ice Creams	1 Bar	60-100
Jell-O Light Pudding Snacks	4 oz.	100
Light Yogurt	6-8 ozs.	100

chapter eleven

Make Fast- Food Fast, Not Fatty

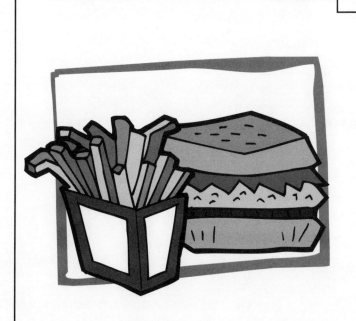

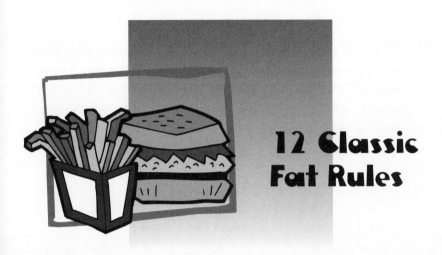

12 Classic Fat Rules

As I told you in the introduction, you'll see that I go over some information more than once. If an important topic falls into more than one category, I'll repeat it. Since everyone gets different things out of what they read, I like to make my points in several different ways. That way, I know that if you don't "get it" in one place, I'm sure you will in another.

Keeping fat intake low is important if you want to be thin. There are a lot of ways to do this and here are the easiest ones to remember:

1. Give low-fat flavors a chance. Your tastebuds may miss the greasy burgers, but they'll get used to eating healthier food if you just let them. You can train your tastebuds to like whatever you tell them to like. It's up to you. Once you are used to eating low-fat foods, food containing higher fat will seem gross and gaggy.

2. Watch portion size. "Low-fat" doesn't mean "low-calorie" and many "reduced fat" products are loaded with sugar. Don't overeat items just because they say "low-fat." Entenmanns' makes a great low-fat donut (I know this to be a fact!) but you can't eat the whole box just because they're low in fat. They are still full of sugar and sugar manufactures fat in your body, too.

3. Read the "ingredients list" on food labels so you don't fall for clever marketing schemes. Chips and crackers that say 'baked not fried' may have been sprayed with oil after they were baked. Look to see how much fat is in your food choice based on the total calorie count. If the fat calories are more than 30% of the total calories, PASS!

4. Try to cut back on the amount of processed foods you eat. These foods tend to be made with hydrogenated or partially hydrogenated vegetable oils and aren't very good for you. They may also be high in sugar and saturated fat, too. Don't forget, processed food is full of chemicals so it will stay fresh in the grocery store longer. Is that really what you want to go into your body???

5. Butter is much better for you than margarine. But, if you must eat margarine, choose one where a liquid vegetable oil is listed before hydrogenated oil. Your best bet is tub margarine which often has "diet margarine"written on the label.

6. Try unsweetened fruit butters or jellies, which don't contain any butter at all, on breads, pancakes & muffins. Apple is the most common flavor that people like and will be found in the jelly sec tion of the market.

7. Grate your cheese instead of adding whole chunks to salads and pastas, or even use grated cheese for grilled cheese sandwiches. You'll be surprised at how much less cheese you'll eat and still not let your tastebuds down.

8. Obey the 'shine rule': If your chips, crackers or bran muffins glisten or leave an oil splotch on a paper bag, chances are they're full of fat so don't eat them!

9. Check the Nutrition Facts label on meats. Ground turkey can be higher in fat than some beef cuts if the turkey is a mix of skin, white & dark meat. Don't always think that because it's red meat, that it will have more fat than other proteins. Poultry can be high in fat, too.

10. Order salad dressing on the side and use a fork to portion it out. Balsamic vinegar makes a great dressing, has almost no calories and is available anywhere. Use it instead of cream dressings whenever you can.

11. Keep track of the amount of saturated fat and total fat in your daily diet by staying away from processed food. Remember: The less saturated fat, the better. If you keep your fats down to 30% of your total daily calorie intake, you will lose weight and maintain the loss without a lot of effort.

12. Don't worry about the fat percentage if you are eating fresh meats, fruits and vegetables. Nature takes care of you and all of those items, for the most part, are well within the 30% rule. If you're eating anything in a box, can or plastic wrap, check the labels. That's where fats are usually hidden!

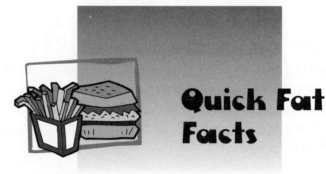

Quick Fat Facts

Once again I remind you, always know exactly what you're eating. Even if it's not good for you, know that you choose to eat it anyway.

Nutrition labels are required on all processed foods. Processed foods are usually the ones that come in boxes, cans or plastic wraps. When you read a label, do you know what that label is telling you? Are you aware of what all the terms mean? If you don't, pay special attention to the "Label Wise" section of this book.

Sometimes we prefer to pretend that we know what the label says so our favorite foods can stay in our grocery carts or lunch tray. Just so your belief files can be more accurate in this area, the terms below are the truth about what you will get when you see the following U.S. government terms on a label:

Fat-Free: The food product must have less than 0.5 grams of fat per serving. Fat content may read "less than 1 gram" or the manufacturer may choose to round the fat content per serving to the nearest gram.

Low-Fat: The food product must have 3 grams or less of fat per serving and the serving must be at least 50 grams total. Let's do the math:
3 fat grams X 9 calories per gram = 27 fat calories

Be sure to see what the total calories are for the 50 gram item to be sure the fat is less than 30% of the total.

Reduced-Fat: Product must have at least 25% less fat than other food just like it and the actual percentage of the reduction must be stated. Hot dogs are a good example for reduced fat. Note that you can have a hot dog that says 95% less fat, but it can still contain 40% to 50% fat. It's just that the hot dog they are comparing it to has 95% more fat by weight than theirs.

Low In Saturated Fat: Food may contain 1 gram or less of saturated fat per serving, and cannot have more than 15% of its calories coming from saturated fat.

Cholesterol Free: The food product must have less than 2 milligrams of cholesterol per serving, and 2 grams or less of saturated fat per serving.

Don't Be Fooled By Labels. Even though this information sounds complete, it is still dangerous if you don't figure out the fat content in your food by yourself. Natural foods are not a problem and you don't need to worry about those. Anything in a package, box, can or bag needs to be calculated. You'll only need to calculate this once, then you'll know what foods to stay away from and which ones you'll need to find alternatives for.

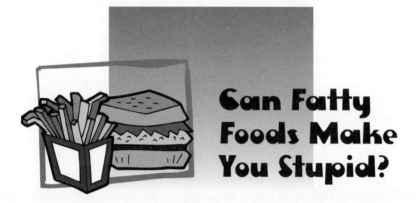

Can Fatty Foods Make You Stupid?

This seems like a silly question but, the truth is...you are what you eat! Since people are getting a lot smarter and not eating as much unhealthy stuff, this has put a big dent in the fast-food industry. A lot of fast-food companies have stepped up to the plate and given us better nutritional value in the meals they offer. Some have even begun to promote their sandwiches as a weight loss option. But, there has been a pretty interesting study which gives medical professionals a lot of reason to believe that greasy hamburgers and other fatty foods can actually make you dumber! Not only will fatty foods make you heavy, now it appears they could reduce your brain function, too!

A study that was done by a dietitian and a psychology professor at the University of Toronto, measured the responses by charting the behavior and activity of 40 rats that they kept on a high-fat diet for six months. Although these were the happiest rats in captivity, having their favorite garbage foods fed to them on a plate every day, the doctors kept a record of how the rats acted and also tested them for learning and memory abilities. By the end of six months, even when these poor little critters were given the simplest tasks to perform, the rats just sat there. Sound familiar? Do you really feel like being productive after eating a double cheeseburger, fries and a coke?

Although the study was done on rats, the researchers decided that what they learned from the rats could also be applied to humans. There is enough similarity, (hard to believe) between a rat and a human's physiologies that we should be concerned.

Now the University of Toronto researchers plan to study humans. They want to know if older people will be smarter and show more mental ability if they make a diet change late in life because of high cholesterol, or fat levels in their body.

If you are someone who has always chowed down on a lot of fast-food, STOP IT! I'm sure, if you start to pay attention to how you feel during classtime, you will soon be aware that your performance throughout the day will improve a bunch when you take more interest in the quality of the food you eat.

Not that we want to follow in the footsteps of our little rat friends, but, if it's not good enough for them...do you really want to eat it?

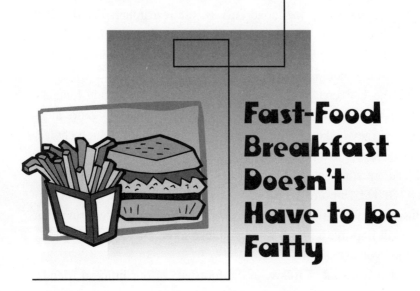

Fast-Food Breakfast Doesn't Have to be Fatty

There is no question that fast food restaurants and the 'need for speed' when it comes to grabbing meals on the run are here to stay. Nationally, Burger King, McDonald's and Hardee's are considered the easiest to find around the country and the most affordable. Unfortunately, if you're not careful with your selections, you could eat the fattiest foods!

Here's a guide on WHAT TO ORDER for the best low-fat breakfasts. We'll get to the other meals in the next section. If it's not inconvenient, the in-home frozen selections may be your best bet and even save you more time. You can even microwave them if a hot breakfast is what you want in the morning.

Take note, McDonalds' Egg McMuffin is THE BEST lowest fat egg sandwich, with only 35% fat. Hardee's is #1 for their low-fat breakfast with their 3 pancake & bacon selection, only 23% fat. But, if you're starting your day with carbs like pancakes, that only leaves you one carb left for later.

So, here the 'skinny' on fast-food breakfast bounty:

BURGER KING	Fat
Croissan'wich with bacon, egg & cheese	60%
Croissan'wich with sausage, egg & cheese	67%
Croissan'wich with ham, egg & cheese	55%
Biscuit with sausage	55%

McDONALD'S	
Egg McMuffin	35%
Bacon, egg & cheese biscuit	53%
Breakfast Burrito	55%
Big Breakfast, eggs, sausage & biscuit	44%
Hash Browns	48%

HARDEE'S	
Rise 'N' Shine biscuit - plain	48%
Ham, egg & cheese biscuit	49%
3 pancakes with 2 bacon strips	23%
Frisco Breakfast ham sandwich	43%

IN HOME - FREEZER SELECTIONS	
Cinnamon-raisin "Big 'n Crusty" bagel	7%
Cinnamon-raisin "Big 'n Crusty" w/cream cheese	30%
Kellogg's Raisin Bran cereal (3/4 cup/1% milk)	14%
Swanson Great Starts sausage biscuit	48%
Pillsbury frozen pancakes w/syrup	27%

RULE OF THUMB: Bacon is better than sausage because it's lower in fat and turkey bacon is better than pork bacon; muffin or biscuit is better than croissant, toast or tortillas is the best of all breads. Use syrup or jelly on pancakes or waffles, but leave off the butter.

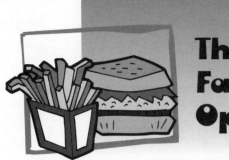

The Best of Your Fast-Food Options

If you're still on the go for lunch and dinner, here are a few lower-fat options. Remember, low-fat does not necessarily mean low-calorie. I have listed items that are under 475 calories so if you know of a sandwich at your favorite restaurant that appears to be lean and is not included in the list, it's most likely to be very high in calories once you add all the catsup, mayo, buns, etc.:

ARBY'S	Fat
Roast Beef Sandwich melt w/Cheddar	19%
Arby-Q Roast Beef Sandwich	15%
Beef 'N Cheddar Sandwich	18%
Giant Roast Beef	28%
Junior Roast Beef	16%
Regular Roast Beef	20%
Super Roast Beef	27%
Chicken Breast Fillet	28%
Grilled Chicken Deluxe	16%
Roast Chicken Club	29%
Grilled Chicken Sandwich	4%

ARBY'S (Continued)	Fat
Light Roast Chicken Deluxe	5%
Light Roast Chicken Salad	5%
Light Roast Turkey Deluxe	5%
Side Salad	3%

BLIMPIE

Roast Beef 6" Sub	12%
Turkey 6" Sub	13%
Grilled Chicken 6" Sub	20%
Club 6" Sub	27%
Blimpie Best 6" Sub	29%
Ham & Swiss 6" Sub	30%
Chicken Fajita	33%

BOSTON MARKET

Rotisserie Turkey Breast	2%
Chicken Sandwich w/o cheese or sauce	7%
Turkey Sandwich w/o cheese or sauce	5%
1/4 White Chicken	5%
Sweet potato; dry	1%
Fruit Salad	1%
Red Beans & Rice	8%
Asst. Vegetables & Corn	5%
Tossed Salad - Fat Free Ranch Dressing	4%
Chicken Chili	11%
Chicken Noodle Soup	17%

BURGER KING
Fat

BK Broiler w/o Mayo	22%

CHICK-FIL-A

Chicken Sandwich	11%
Chicken Club Sandwich	28%
Chicken-N-Strips	30%
Chicken Salad Sandwich	12%
Hearty Breast of Chicken Soup (cup)	9%
Chargrilled Chicken Garden Salad	8%
Chick-N-Strips Salad	26%
Chicken Caesar Salad	15%

DAIRY QUEEN

Grilled Chicken Filet Sandwich	29%

JACK-IN-THE-BOX

Chicken Teriyaki Bowl	6%
Fajita Pita	29%

LONG JOHN SILVER'S

Side Salad	0%
Corn Cobbette	6%
Rice Pilaf	18%
Flavorbaked Chicken	27%
Flavorbaked Fish	28%
Flavorbaked Chicken Sandwich	31%

McDONALD'S
Fat

Chicken McGrill w/o Mayo	18%

TACO BELL

Bean Burrito	29%
Grilled Chicken Burrito	30%
Chicken Soft Taco	30%

WENDY'S

Grilled Chicken Caesar	30%
Plain Baked Potato	0%
Chili w/o cheese	29%
Garden Ranch Chicken Pita	33%
Grilled Chicken Sandwich	23%

If you have the need for sweets, Dairy Queen is the national favorite for low-fat treats. However, sugar is still a factor and calories range from 60 to 320 per serving:

(* under 100 calories)

DAIRY QUEEN	Fat
Lemon Freez'r	0%*
Misty Slush	0%
Starkiss	0%*
Strawberry Misty Cooler	0%
Vanilla Orange Bar	0%*
Strawberry Breeze	0%
Yogurt Strawberry Sundae	2%
Yogurt Cone - regular	1%
Vanilla Cone - small	26%
Ice Cream Sandwich	20%

Other chains like TCBY and Yogurt-To-Go have fat-free and low-fat options for dessert as well. Check out your local store, but stay away from the ice cream and topping selections.

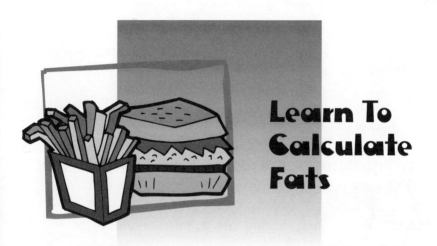

Learn To Calculate Fats

Did you know that a 1999 opinion poll showed that 17% of the American public thought that the healthiest diet they could eat meant that they would be eating zero fat? Thank goodness that achieving a zero-fat diet is almost impossible for the average person, since being completely fat-free would kill you!

As you have heard me say throughout this book, your goal is to keep the amount of fat you eat each day under 30 percent of your total calorie count. If you're eating fresh fruits and vegetables, or fresh meats from the butcher department, you don't need to worry about the fat content you're getting. Generally speaking, nature provides well for you by not putting more than 30 percent fat in anything it creates.

The only fats you need to be concerned about are those found in packaged, boxed or shrink-wrapped products. Just to be sure you're not overdoing it, check the labels on those items you eat all the time. Once you become an expert label-reader, nobody will ever be able to trick you into eating high-fat stuff again!

This is what you need to do when checking out your labels:

1. Find the total number of fat grams per serving on the package.

2. Multiply the number of fat grams times 9 to equal the number of fat calories per serving.

3. Divide the number of fat calories by the total calories per serving. This will give you the percentage of fat for that item.

EXAMPLE: A single hotdog has a total calorie count of 140 calories and contains 11 fat grams;

11 fat grams x 9 calories per gram = 99 fat calories.
99 fat calories divided by 140 total calories for the hotdog equals 71% fat!

Another fat source, trans-fatty acids, are the bad fats we talked about in hydrogenated or partially hydrogenated domestic oils, and are more harmful to your health than saturated fats.

A 1999 study showed that babies born to mothers who ate large amounts of trans-fatty acids (partially hydrogenated domestic oils) during their pregnancy showed metabolic abnormalities, meaning the baby's metabolism was already very slow. When a baby's metabolism is slow, it will limit their ability to grow and develop correctly.

If something contains hydrogenated domestic oils it will clearly say so on the product label. Read your labels and avoid those products as much as you can.

chapter twelve

Eat For Your Body, Too

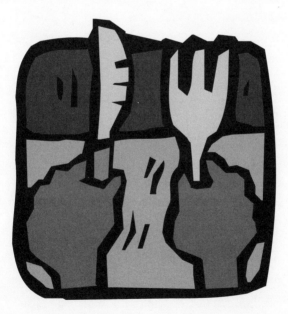

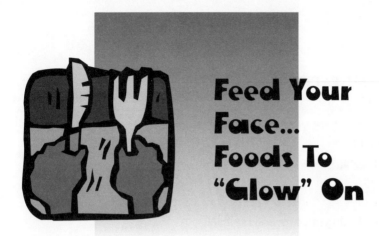

Feed Your Face... Foods To "Glow" On

We all want to look great and just by eating certain healthy foods, we can look better. Nutrition is just as important for your face as it is for your body.

It is well-documented that vitamin deficiencies lead to dry flaky skin, hair loss, and brittle nails. Iron deficiency, which is more common among women in their 20s' than in their teens, can leave complexions pale and drawn. Zinc shortages can cause flaky and rash-prone skin, and leave you open to get more colds. Taking vitamin and mineral supplements can ensure you're getting all the nutritional elements you need if eating regular, balanced meals is too hard for you.

Here are a few 'skin essential foods' and what they will do to help you have a "fit face:"

BETA-CAROTENE
Sources: Orange colored vegetables and fruits (carrots, sweet potatoes, squash, cantaloupe, apricots) and spinach.
Benefit: Considered to help ward-off cancer and keep skin cells young.

BIOTIN
Sources: Cheese, eggs, peanut butter.
Benefit: Essential for strong hair and nails. Don't eat too much of these because of their high fat content. One serving per day of your choice is ideal.

ESSENTIAL FATTY ACIDS

Sources: Cooking oils (corn, olive, safflower) and Essential Fatty Acid supplements.
Benefit: Keeps skin moist and supple.

IRON
Sources: Red meat, broccoli, spinach.
Benefit: Deficiency can cause itchy, pale skin and fatigue.

SELENIUM
Sources: Meat, seafood, milk, vegetables, whole grains.
Benefit: May reduce sun damage and protect against non-melanoma skin cancers.

VITAMIN A
Sources: Eggs, butter, liver.
Benefit: High doses have helped prevent recurrences of skin cancer. Deficiency can cause dry flaky skin.

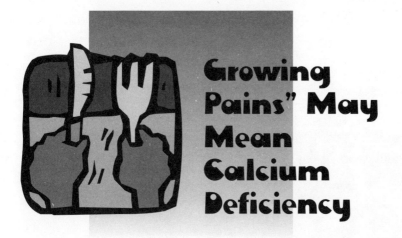

"Growing Pains" May Mean Calcium Deficiency

It's not unusual for new dieters or growing teenagers to complain of leg cramps. These are also sometimes called, "growing pains." You can keep leg cramping to a minimum if you eat calcium-rich foods such as low-fat dairy products, kale and broccoli at some point each day. If you're pretty good about eating dairy products like yogurt, milk and cheese, you will probably have much fewer leg cramps than the average person.

Potassium is another mineral that will help eliminate leg cramps. Apples and bananas are both great sources of potassium before bedtime. You will also find potassium in sweet potatoes and many fruits like figs, cantaloupe, kiwi, and papaya.

If leg cramps have been bugging you for awhile, you may try to exercise a little more. When you stretch and warm-up your muscles on a regular basis, they get a better blood flow and don't tend to cramp as much. If you don't exercise at all now, don't confuse the soreness that can follow the beginning of an exercise program with leg cramps. If you've got muscles that haven't been used much lately, they'll hurt a little for a day or two. Once you keep up the workouts, the hurt will go away and a terrific new energy will take its place!

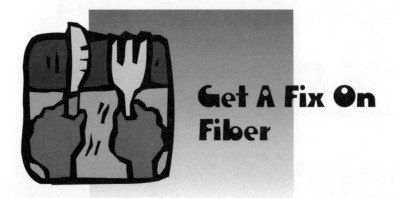

Get A Fix On Fiber

At this stage of the game, as a kid, you're probably pretty unaware of how important something like fiber is to your diet. Most kids are under the impression that diseases and health problems will never happen to them. But, the body you have right now is the only one you'll ever have so you need to take care of it the best way you can.

You want to be sure to get enough fiber in your diet because it helps digestion and lowers cancer risks - especially colon cancer. Since I promote a low starchy-carbohydrate eating program, sometimes it's hard knowing what to eat in order to fill your daily fiber requirements.

Here are 10 helpful hints to add fiber and flavor to your diet:

1. **Eat meats on top of grains.** Chicken, fish and beef dishes are far more interesting when served on a bed of lentils, barley, couscous or whole-wheat rice.

2. **Eat your citrus fruits, don't juice them.** The white part of the fruit rind is a great source of fiber. Peel grapefruits and oranges and leave some of the rind in tact. Doctors feel that soluble fibers such as those found in apples, peaches,

pears, oranges and grapefruits can help lower and may even prevent high cholesterol levels and high blood pressure. Eating citrus fruits also lowers your chance for heart disease and diabetes.

3. **Ask mom to add wheat bran to chicken or seafood breading.** Shaking one 1/2 cup of wheat bran into breading can boost fiber-poor meals without a lot of extra calories, which is good for the whole family.

4. **Add vegetables to entreé dishes.** Toss broccoli, spinach or peppers onto pizza, or mix them with your favorite pasta dish. Scrambled eggs or omelets taste a lot better when made with chopped veggies inside. Try it!

5. **Eat breakfast cereals (with limitation!) as a snack, too.** If you like cereal, breakfast doesn't have to be the only time you eat it. A low-fat, healthy cereal can take the edge off while waiting for the next meal time. And, if you have a hard time sleeping at night, a bowl of cereal rich in high fiber will often do the trick to help you sleep better. Remember, cereal still counts as one of your starch portions for the day, so don't go crazy. Just try and eat cereals with a healthy fiber content - it will say so on the box.

6. **Eat your potatoes baked, not mashed or fried.** A baked potato with the skin left on is a huge improvement in terms of fiber over a regular potato prepared any other way. Sweet potatoes are even better because they have much more flavor than a regular potato and require less stuff on them to

make them taste good. In addition, sweet potatoes are a wonderful source of valuable nutrients like beta-carotene.

7. **Make your French toast with whole grain bread.** Whole grain pancake mixes are also available at the supermarket.

8. **Have a spinach salad instead of the usual lettuce.** Plain iceberg lettuce is fairly low in fiber. If you're not much of a spinach fan, that doesn't mean you won't like it in a salad. Chop the leaves up along with other fresh vegetables and mix regular lettuce with them, if you're not sure. You'll be surprised how good it tastes.

9. **Snack on dried fruit or use them as toppings for yogurt both regular yogurt and frozen.** Dried fruit is an excellent source of fiber, vitamins, iron, potassium and beta-carotene, however, it is also very high in sugar and calorie content, so don't go crazy with it... use it sparingly.

10. **Chow down on chili.** Chili beans are a wonderful source of fiber. And when it's made with meat and zesty sauces, it becomes a great source of high protein, too. Canned or cooked fried beans can also be added to your favorite stews or soups for an extra fiber boost.

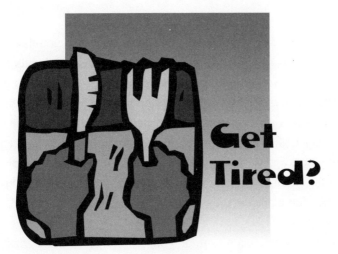

Get Tired?

If the afternoon snoozies are a problem for you, don't believe the commercials you see on TV that tell you to have a candy bar when you need a boost of energy. I bet you didn't know that eating too much refined sugar, which is what is in your average candy bar, will actually make you more tired and have less energy. It's true! You might get a quick energy jolt, but you'll come back to earth pretty fast and usually with a heavier bump that can even make you sleepy!

Here's another tid-bit for your science project so you know the real reason: Diets high in sugar cause the pancreas to secrete too much insulin which actually leads to low blood sugar, or 'hypoglycemia.' Pretty technical stuff, but I want you to at least keep up with the rats!

Anyway, if you feel your energy draining away late mornings and afternoons, and experience mood swings where you're cranky or really tired, your body may be experiencing low blood sugar. Taking care of this problem will not happen overnight, but eating less sugar, more protein and fiber like whole grains and fruits, will soon make a difference.

If you get tired after you eat lunch as opposed to late afternoons, you may be eating too much fat and not enough vegetables or carbohydrates. You also want to make sure that this happens pretty often before you make a lot of dietary changes. You don't want to change your eating too much only to find that your sleepy condition is because you have a boring afternoon class and has nothing to do with your eating habits!

Food plays an important part in energizing you. Here's a little more science: In two human studies, people who ate more fats and less carbohydrates were less alert than those who ate less fats. The people eating more fat also had a harder time concentrating on tasks that required longer attention spans, and, were less cheerful with the people they worked with. (See, we're just like our rat friends!) People on a high-fat diet said they felt a drop in their ability to pay attention about 2-1/2 hours after eating.

For now, you may want to trade your hamburger and fries or ham & cheese sandwich for a piece of grilled chicken and a side salad or beef & vegetable stir-fry. Then, watch your afternoon energy increase. Be your own science project and conduct good eating tests on yourself. I know you'll love your findings!

If you are constantly tired, and you don't eat many nuts, legumes, dried beans, or non-citrus fruits like bananas, cherries or plums, you may be lacking the trace mineral boron. Boron is necessary for you to keep alert and energized. You are what you eat. If you start to eat energizing boron-packed food again, you'll be back to feeling great and awake in no-time.

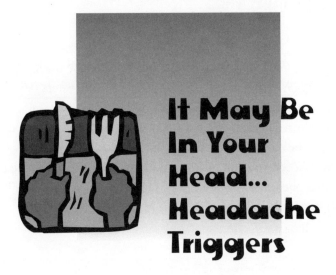

It May Be In Your Head... Headache Triggers

Headaches are never any fun but, be prepared that you may have a headache or two when you start making changes in your eating habits. Since you probably eat a lot of starchy carbohydrates right now, you could go through what food experts lovingly call "carbohydrate withdrawal." Carbohydrates are what your body turns into glucose or sugar for energy. Anytime you eat less carbs than what your body is used to, the lessening of the sugar your body now makes can cause you to get a headache for a day or two.

If 'carbohydrate withdrawal headaches' should happen to you, aspirin (or whatever your parents usually have you take for headache pain) will generally do the trick. If you are currently a high-carbohydrate and starch eater, try to cut back slowly so that your body isn't hit too hard with the change all at one time. Don't go from eight servings of bread to two immediately - cut back a little each day until your body is comfortable with the food adjustment.

Uh-Oh...Chocolate may be a problem, too! Sorry to break the news to you if you already know you're a chocoholic, but it has been proven that chocolate can cause migraine headaches. A study was conducted in England with people who got a lot of headaches. 50% of the patients were asked to eat peppermint-laced chocolate and the other 50% ate what the people THOUGHT was chocolate, but was actually made of carob and peppermint. Within one day, 88% of the chocolate eaters developed headaches and 100% of the carob eaters were headache-free.

This doesn't mean you can't have chocolate anymore. It just means that you need to be responsible about the amount of treats you allow yourself every day. When you don't take things like chocolate for granted and stop eating it all the time, you'll be surprised at what a special treat it can become. And, with less headache!

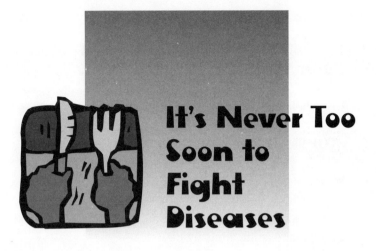

It's Never Too Soon to Fight Diseases

As we enter into a new century, we hope to find cures for many diseases but more and more diseases that were unheard of 20 years ago, seem to be affecting all of us.

Cancer research and cures have come a long way, but this ugly disease seems to touch everyone. If you don't know someone who has been affected by cancer already, you probably will, in some way. Unfortunately, it may be sooner than you think.

Simple changes in your eating habits and lifestyle can make all the difference in keeping you healthy. Start now and you're giving yourself a much better chance at a disease-free life!

Here are a few tips:

1. Eat a diet rich in vegetables, fruits, and grains. You should eat at least 5-9 servings of fruit and veggies daily.

2. Eat plenty of carrots, spinach, cabbage, cauliflower and broccoli, which are rich in beta-carotene. Sweet potatoes also contain a rich supply of beta-carotene.

3. Try to have a lot of tomatoes, watermelon, red peppers, and strawberries.

4. Use whole grains whenever possible.

5. **STOP SMOKING**.

6. Wear a sunscreen of at least SPF 15 when you're outside.

7. Young ladies should check their breasts monthly for lumps and get regular examinations by their doctor.

8. Drink no more than 2 cups of coffee daily.

9. Stay away from fried, cured and smoked foods like bacon, ham and hotdogs. If you eat these foods, have a glass of orange juice, rich in vitamin C to lessen stomach problems.

10. Cut back in fats (for weight loss and health).

11. Don't automatically salt your food. Most prepared foods have enough salt in them already. Fresh foods may need some additional spices.

12. Eat foods with plenty of vitamin A, C, and E and take an antioxidant. Antioxidants help fight the free radicals in the air that we are exposed to through sun, fumes and other pollutants.

13. Stay positive and keep your mind healthy.

If you're not a big fruit and vegetable person...YOU CAN BE! I'm sure there are a lot of things you eat now that you never liked when you were very little. I remember going to Chinese restaurants with my parents when I was about 7 years old and would only eat fried rice because I hated Chinese food. Now I love it. Many people are surprised to learn that American and cheddar are not the only cheeses you can buy. Don't laugh. I know many people who have never had anything other than

American cheese because "they already know they won't like anything else!" Can you imagine how much people limit themselves when they predetermine what they will and will not like? The sad thing is, this kind of attitude usually trickles over into other areas of their life, too.

Food will become more of an enjoyment and less of a fear if you experiment a little and try new things. You may think I'm crazy, but you can actually learn to like foods that are good for you! Of course, you can't learn to enjoy what you refuse to try. But, training your tastebuds is possible and enjoyable if you JUST DO IT!

If fruits or vegetables have never been your 'thing,' start slowly. Have some kind of fruit or veggie item every-other-day until you find the ones that you enjoy eating most often. Some people start eating vegetables by having vegetable soup. That's a good place to start. You get a little of quite a few veggie items in a single serving.

How your food is cooked is important, too. Some mom's overcook vegetables until they're limp and flavorless. If that sounds familiar, try ordering steamed vegetables sometime when you're out to dinner so you can taste what they're supposed to taste like and see if you don't change your mind. You may be surprised at how great they taste. Or, maybe you'd like them better raw. The options are unlimited - you just need to keep an open mind and be willing to experiment.

Diseases can be fought the best with a combination of good food and good thinking. Negative energy creates all kinds of negative activity in your body. Remember, your mind tells your body how it's supposed to act and feel. If your mind is full of negative thoughts about how weak you are, or is always thinking about all the things you can't do, how is your body going to feel strong and healthy?

The picture you visualized when you began reading this book was of a happy, healthy and thin person. Now, it's up to you to live up to the image you have created for yourself. You have the power inside you to look and feel any way you want. It's completely up to you. If you live the lifestyle that you think the image in your picture would live, and don't accept anything but the best out of yourself, you'll be everything you want to be...and more.

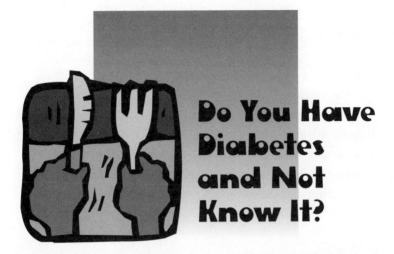

Do You Have Diabetes and Not Know It?

This section may not apply to you, but it's one that is important because diabetes is a disease that greatly affects overweight people. In adults, Type II non-insulin dependent (meaning you don't need to take insulin shots every day) diabetes usually develops slowly. Risk factors include a family history of diabetes, being over 30 years of age, and being overweight. Unfortunately, diabetes is growing at alarming rates amongst our nation's teens, too.

If diabetes runs in your family or if you have some of the symptoms listed here, speak to your parents about it and have them check with your doctor. Diabetes in young people is sometimes overlooked and may be hidden behind an overweight condition. But, it could also be an explanation for overactive sugar cravings you may have. If you think this might apply to you, ask your doctor to test you. Identifying a possible medical problem will certainly help make your weight loss efforts a little easier.

The symptoms of diabetes include:

- Feeling tired
- Blurred vision
- Dry, itchy skin
- Increased hunger and thirst
- Increased urination
- Tingling or loss of feeling in hands and feet
- Non-healing infections of skin, vagina, and/or bladder
- Vaginal yeast infections

Many times people show no symptoms when diabetes is still present and diagnosed. See your doctor if you suspect either you or a family member may have diabetes. Once diagnosed, diabetes can be managed with frequent monitoring of blood sugar, diet and medication. Insulin may not even be needed. You'll always feel better when you know for sure.

chapter thirteen

Eating At School

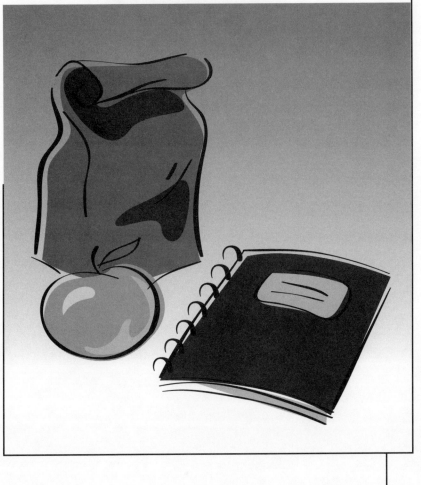

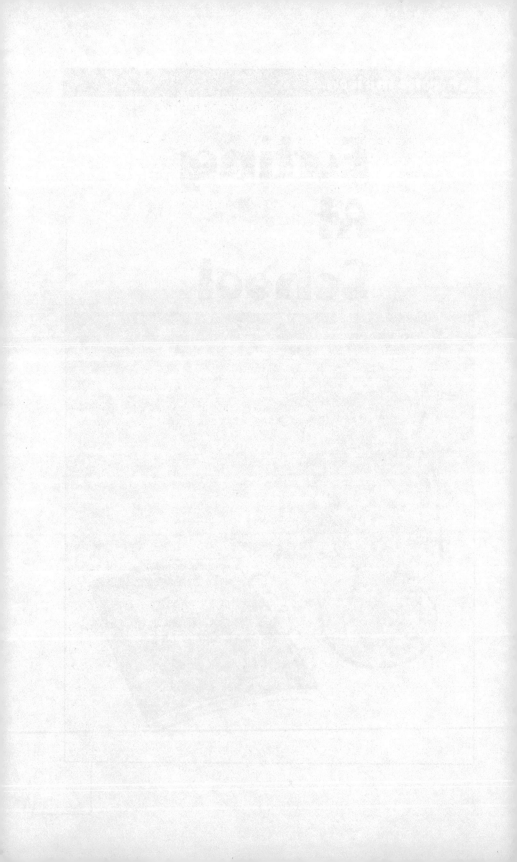

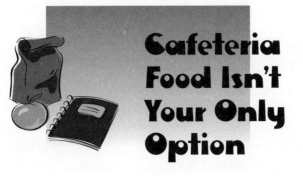

Cafeteria Food Isn't Your Only Option

Isn't it amazing that most schools teach some form of nutrition in their health classes when they certainly don't "practice what they preach" in the cafeteria. It's no wonder that kids today are growing by leaps and bounds (not only up, but out!) when they're not offered good-tasting food that's also good for them.

Most schools offer high-fat "mystery meals" with weird sauces and yucky meat that drives students to the snack counter where they end up creating their lunch from a large selection of chips, cookies and other nutritionally poor, high carbohydrate items.

So, what can you do about this? Bring your lunch! OK, I know that sounds like a pain, but it's really not a big deal to take some sliced turkey or barbecued chicken with you each day. Even a can of water-packed chicken or tuna gives you lots of protein without a lot of trouble. If you have access to a microwave oven, you can always make soup or bring in a light TV-style dinner. Healthy Choice, Weight Watchers and Lean Cuisine all make good tasting, low-fat meals that are certainly better than most cafeteria options. You don't have to get up early to make sandwiches, just take fresh cut (not packaged) deli meat with you. You're better off without the bread anyway. Dribble on a little mustard, wrap the meat around a quarter dill pickle slice or celery, and you're in business!

Most cafeterias offer fresh fruit, yogurt or cottage cheese and even a salad bar, so give those a try, too. But, go lightly on the salad dressing, or even keep a bottle of balsamic vinegar in your locker. If your school serves hamburgers, try eating the burger patty without the bun. The same thing goes for chicken or any luncheon meat sandwich. Use mustard or catsup instead of mayonnaise. If you're lucky enough to have a fast-food company such as Taco Bell on your school campus, have grilled chicken or a steak burrito. Tortillas are a light, fat-free option to eating bread.

It's important for brain function and mental alertness that you are properly nourished when you're at school. Most kids get at least one-third of their daily nutrition from school cafeterias, so your selections are important if you are eating on campus.

If eating at school is more hassle than you can handle, then be sure to have a good breakfast in the morning and a healthy snack as soon as you get home. Don't overdo the afternoon snack if dinner tends to be eaten early. You certainly don't have the option of going all day without food, so you're going to have to come up with some workable solution to this problem.

Protein bars are another option as long as you don't pick the ones that are loaded with carbs. Be sure that the bars you pick have at least 15 grams of protein in them with a minimum amount of fat. Fruit is another alternative although you still need a little protein to help get you through the day. Next time mom goes to the market, join her. See if anything strikes your fancy if school food is simply out of the question.

chapter fourteen

It's Cool to Be Smart

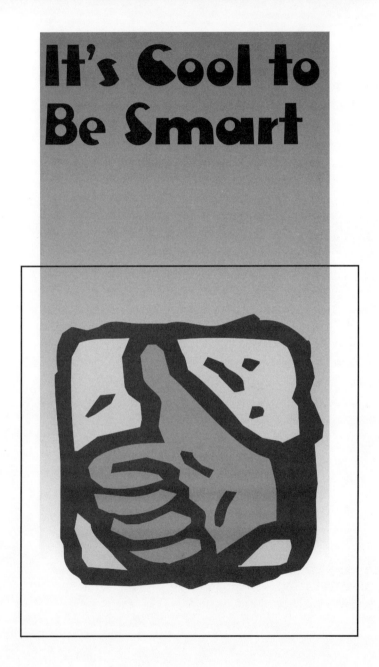

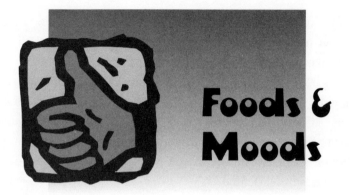

Foods &
Moods

Next time you're in a really stinky mood, think of your head as being one giant lemon! It's sour, full of acid and nobody ever wants too much of it!

I'm sure you'll agree that the foods you eat affect how you feel. When you know you haven't eaten very well, your body tells you in the form of stomach aches, gas, nervousness, lack of energy or just plain feeling yucky. If your body is lacking something, it will tell you in the form of cravings. The connection between you and the food you eat is very big.

Food also can play a very big role in controlling your emotions. Children who are generally pretty hyper-active need to stay away from a lot of sugar because sweets only makes their condition worse. The sugar energizes them more. For some, food is also used for comfort when they feel unhappy. Their emotional files have been programmed to tell them that tasty treats become a type of reward to help lift their spirits.

Even though we can create an emotional link between ourselves and what we eat, the fact is, there is a real chemical link happening at the same time. Your body is one big chemical machine. The food you eat is made up of nutrients that create a bunch of chemicals too. When the chemical balance in your body doesn't mix well with the chemical balance of the food you eat, you're not a happy camper. Depending on how much your balance becomes out-of-whack will dictate how unhappy or uncomfortable you may become.

Stress is a condition that affects the body the most. When stress hits, you're more likely to crave carbohydrates like pasta or bread than anything else. Carbs like these trigger the release of serotonin, a brain-calming agent. Since these kinds of foods are higher in calories than protein, and require a fair amount of energy burn to use them up in our body, weight gain isn't far behind.

While your brain may be getting calmer, the carbohydrates are causing your body's blood-sugar levels to shoot up when you first eat them, then plunge back down as they get digested in the body. This creates even more stress because the adrenal glands are more stimulated. Your blood sugar levels sometimes spike up as much as 150% from sugary treats, causing heart rate increases of 33 beats per-minute. Now you know why you may not feel so great about an hour after you eat a donut!

Stress isn't a bug or virus that we catch. It's just the way our bodies respond on the inside to events happening on the outside. This kind of upset can be caused by a zillion different things: Danger, feeling like you have so much to do that you can't handle it all, or even being afraid to speak in front of your whole class. Along with an increase in food cravings to calm us down, the different systems in our bodies are greatly affected when we're stressed.

Here's a little more information from a 'science project' point-of-view. It's all a little technical but I want you to really understand the kind of impact that upset has on your body and all the different organs and systems that are affected: In addition to adrenaline, the nervous system lets off a bunch of stuff. The brain then sends a message to the body telling it to lessen the blood flow to the digestive system so it's harder to process the foods you eat. The release of adrenaline and the neurotransmitters affects your cardio-vascular system so your heart beats faster and your blood pressure goes up. Your breathing will become faster, too.

When all your systems are not working right, your digestive system slows even more as stomach acid increases. This causes you to feel heartburn and indigestion. Because the blood flow is less, the lower digestive system slows down, too. This creates poor digestion of the food you're eating.

When stress hits, your body's immune system is greatly affected. That means your infection fighting cells, which are your antibodies and T-lymphocytes, are not being created properly so you become more likely to catch colds, flu, and other infections.

Only you can control your stress. If stress doesn't bother you very often, the few times it does is not a big deal. Even though your body will go through the same process I just explained, it will quickly return to normal. But, if stress is an everyday event, the assault on your body becomes a daily event too so, STOP IT!

It is amazing that doctors feel the majority of all their patient's visits are for health-related problems that have been caused by stress. Since stress sends off so many chemical reactions in the body, cravings for the wrong kinds of food becomes a daily part of your life and weight gain is right there, knocking on your door.

Turning to food when you're upset or uptight doesn't solve any problems. The only thing that will most likely happen is that you'll gain a few additional pounds while you're 'eating your heart out.' Nothing will solve your dilemmas other than tackling them head on. Using food to comfort you may help you feel better for a few minutes, but whatever is troubling you hasn't gone away and is still there, staring you in the face. So, face it. You can't hide behind food forever. When you learn to accept life's challenges and take them on, one at a time, you'll find that your stress level goes down a lot.

You've already taken the first step in creating a healthy, new relationship with your mind and body. Now that you're mind knows what to do, your body will have no other option but to follow!

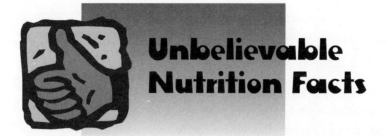

Unbelievable Nutrition Facts

Did you know?

• Children need 1 ½ to 2 times more protein per pound of body weight than adults. Babies need 3-times more.

• Vitamin B1 can help fight air and seasickness.

• Eating food containing too much artificial flavors, colors, MSG and other additives interferes with the function of the immune system.

• 80% of American women are deficient in calcium.

• One cigarette destroys up to 100 mg. of vitamin C.

• Raw peanuts contain enzyme inhibitors that make it difficult for your body to digest protein.

• Water softeners create an unhealthy increase to your daily salt intake, so drink bottled water instead.

• Pasta packed in cellophane or with large cellophane windows, lose their nutrients.

- Blueberries, blackberries, and red cabbage are actually better for you if you cook them.

- Yellow and red onions, red grapes, and broccoli are rich in quercetin, which has been discovered as an anti-cancer agent that can suppress malignant cells before they form tumors.

- Olive oil is one of the best heart disease-fighting natural foods available.

- Avoiding black coffee may help you avoid cancer of the esophagus.

- There may be a connection between toothpaste and bowel diseases such as colitis, Crohn's disease and irritable bowel syndrome. Rinse well and do not swallow the toothpaste.

- New studies show that non-smokers live eighteen years longer than smokers.

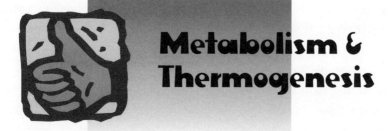

Metabolism & Thermogenesis

Even though some of the information I've put in this book doesn't directly deal with your eating habits or behavior changes, I think it's important that you know how your body works. The more you know about the way your body functions, the easier it is to understand why you need to get your head and your body under control as soon as you can. Even though you're the guy that has to control what you eat, some of your weight problem may not be your fault at all. An overweight condition may genetically run in your family, or your parents may not understand about how important good nutrition is. No matter what the reason, anything is 'fixable.'

Weight loss isn't just about food. It's also about how your body uses the food you eat and if you help it along with other energizing options like exercise. The only way to lose weight is to speed up your metabolism so your body can burn-off excess fat and calories. If you don't elevate your metabolism higher than it is right now, then you'll stay the same size. It's just that simple. If you currently exercise, then you need to exercise more in order for you to raise your metabolism to a more productive, weight loss-oriented level.

Metabolism is the process where the body eats up oxygen to make enough energy so that your brain, heart, lungs and other parts of your body work properly. When the metabolism is slow, your body processes things slower. When it comes to your weight, the slower your body processes the foods you eat, the easier it is to gain.

Some people are born with faster metabolisms than others but, as we get older, metabolism can slow down all by itself. Too much dieting, bad eating habits, medical conditions, prescriptions drugs and even smoking affects how fast your metabolism works. The healthier you eat and the more you exercise, the better your metabolism energizes your body.

THERMOGENESIS, means the generation of heat or "burning up calories." Thermogenesis is a normal body process like digestion. The purpose of thermogenesis is to burn up the calories your body doesn't need. Being overweight, or obese, occurs mostly when thermogenesis is not working right, or your metabolism is too slow. When thermogenesis isn't happening and your metabolism slows way down, the body is forced to deal with all the excess calories itself, so it just stores them all over as fat.

Ever wonder why some people stay thin while their body burns off excess calories no matter what they eat, yet other people seem to put on extra pounds and inches just by looking at a hot fudge sundae? Scientists have been wondering about this for years, too. Even though we weren't really "born to be fat," some of us do have genes that almost force us to stay in an overweight condition. This is not impossible to overcome, but it does make your weight loss efforts a little more challenging.

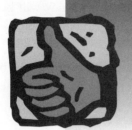

What is a Plateau?

Everyone hits them, and everyone HATES them! The miserable "plateau" is that weight level you hit and can't get off for at least two-weeks. Your body has a memory. As you gained your weight in the first place, your body remembers each weight level you stopped on. As you start to lose weight now, your body may stop on the same levels you held as you were gaining. Make sense?

If you were 120 pounds for awhile, then you gained weight and stopped gaining when you reached 140 pounds, your body remembers these weight levels. If you eventually hit 160 pounds and started to lose weight, you can pretty much bet that you'll hit plateaus at the 140 pound and 120 pound levels.

Don't mix short pauses in weight reduction with "plateaus." You may not lose pounds every single day. You may only see the scale going down once a week. These on-again-off-again- stops in weight loss don't need to be dealt with by extreme "plateau breaking" measures. You may just be trading pounds.

You only want to use of one of my suggested plateau breakers when you've really hit a plateau, or they won't work for you after awhile. Your body slows down with repetition. That's why I want you to rotate your foods and not eat the same things every day. If you use one of my plateau-breaking suggestions every week, pretty soon they will become part of your regular routine and the plateau breaker will no longer work for you.

Here's the deal: If you have stayed at the same weight level for two or more weeks, then you can try one of the following ways to break your weight plateau. Any one will help jump-start your metabolism into burning more fat:

1. Three Days, No Starchy Carbohydrates. Eat only vegetables, proteins, fruits and dairy for three days. Don't eat any like breads or pastas during this time. Try to stay away from apples also if you pick this plateau-breaker since apples are high in carbohydrates, too. Use this option for only 3 days, period. On day four you can go back to eating two starch servings every day and your weight level should finally drop.

2. Eat Only Apples. This is extreme, but it does work. Eat nothing but apples for one day. When the carbohydrates in apples are your body's only source of energy for the day, they will act as a cleansing process and boost your weight loss again.

3. Eat Anything. That's right, go crazy for one day ONLY. Since most of us eat about the same things all the time, it's not unusual for your body to get used to the foods you eat. When you go crazy for one day and eat items you would usually try not to eat like pizza, ice cream, chips, and stuff, the difference in the food you are eating for one day, along with your change in eating pattern will shock your body into losing. Because the things you're eating for this one day are so different from the ones you eat most of the time, it forces your metabolism to speed up so it can work off these unusual items. Once your metabolism gets cookin,' your weight loss follows!

Plateau-breaker number three IS NOT your permission ticket to binge eating! This way of breaking a plateau is only to be used when the plateau you're on has lasted for at least two to three weeks. Do not use this "eat everything" practice on a regular basis or you'll gain weight faster than you can imagine.

REMEMBER: If you treat every short-term stop in your weight as a plateau and use one of these methods on a regular basis, that plateau-breaker won't work when you really need it. Try and break each plateau you hit with good eating patterns first. If that doesn't work, then you may use one of these methods to help.

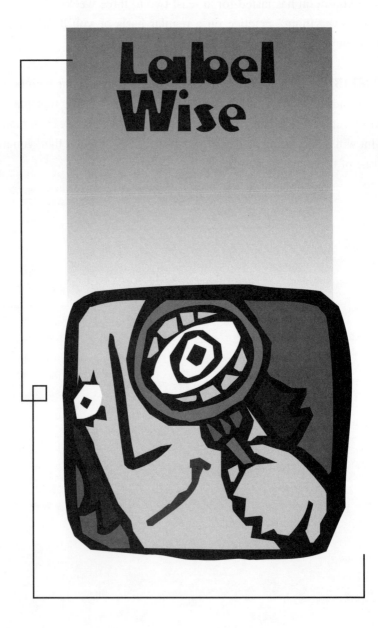

chapter fifteen

Label Wise

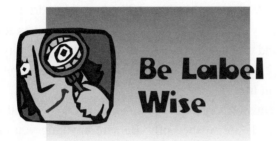

Be Label Wise

Reading labels will help you make smart food choices. Everything you need to know about a packaged food is written on the label. So, READ THE LABEL! Don't go by the "light," "lean," "low-fat" message on the front. Read the serving size, calorie count and fat content, too. Labels are designed to sell products. Manufacturers make their labels in such a way that it grabs your attention and makes you want to buy it. Fancy words like "light" and "diet" sell products, but they can mislead you into thinking you're buying something that's healthy for you when it may not be. When you read the fat and calories per serving in the nutrition section and know that you're eating 30% or less in fat, then you've got nothing to worry about.

I keep harping on you to give up processed and packaged foods. I do that because I know it's really hard to control the amount of sugar, fats, sodium, additives, and preservatives that's packed into that stuff. I'm the first one to say you can't stay away from packaged items completely, but you can cut down. Fresh meats, fruits and vegetables will always give your body better metabolic energy plus...they just taste better!

No matter what the item is, you always want your food to be fresh. Check the expiration date. Dairy products are especially tricky because there is nothing worse than having bad milk or cheese. Always check the expiration date - even if it's in your own refrigerator. If your house is like mine, the new milk can get put in front of a carton I bought last week. Once the new milk is gone, the older milk is too old to drink.

I know there is a lot of stuff for you to remember when it comes to eating healthy and taking care of yourself the right way. Pretty soon, all the things you're reading about in this book will become habit, just like everything else in life.

Wash your fruits & vegetables before you eat them so all the pesticides and chemicals are washed off. Be sure anything you open from your pantry that says, "refrigerate after opening" gets put into the refrigerator. And, **READ YOUR LABELS** so you always know exactly what you're eating.

Even though this may sound like a lot to remember right now, don't worry about it. When you're not sure what to do, you can always look back in this book as a reminder. Just think "good health" and most of your actions will come naturally like washing your hands. The healthier your body is, and the better you treat it, the faster it will get rid of your excess weight.

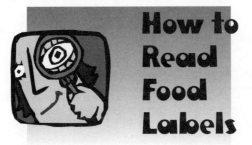

How to Read Food Labels

HOW TO READ THE NEW FOOD LABELS

SERVING SIZE
Is your serving the same size as the one on the label? If you eat double the serving size listed, you need to double the nutrient and calorie values. If you eat half the serving size shown here, cut the nutrient and calorie values in half.

CALORIES
Are you overweight? Cut back a little on the calories! Look here to see how a serving of food adds to your daily total. A 5'4", 138-lb active woman needs about 2,200 calories each day. A 5'10", 174-lb active man needs about 2,900 calories. How about you?

TOTAL CARBOHYDRATES
When you cut down on fat, you can eat more carbohydrates. Carbohydrates are in foods like bread, potatoes, fruits and vegetables. Choose these often! They give you more nutrients than sugars like soda pop and candy.

DIETARY FIBER
Grandmother called it "roughage," but her advice to eat more is still up to date! That goes for both soluble and insoluble kinds of dietary fiber. Fruits, vegetables, whole-grain foods, beans and peas are all good sources and can reduce the risk of heart disease and cancer.

PROTEIN
Most Americans get more protein than they need. Where there is animal protein, there is also fat and cholesterol. Eat small servings of lean meat, fish and poultry. Use skim or low-fat milk, yogurt and cheese. Try vegetable proteins like beans, grains and cereals.

VITAMINS AND MINERALS
Your goal here is 100 percent of each for the day. One food cannot do it all. Let a combination of foods add up to a winning score.

Nutrition Facts

Serving Size 1 Bar(41g)
Servings Per Container 6

Calories 170   Calories from Fat 45

	%Daily Value*
Total Fat 5g	8%
Saturated Fat 2g	10%
Cholesterol 0g	0%
Sodium 160mg	6%
Potassium 40mg	0%
Total Carbohydrates 16g	5%
Dietary Fiber 0g	0%
Sugars 6g	
Protein 15g	30%

Calcium 12%	Iron	8%

Not a significant source of Vitamin A and Vitamin C

*Percent Daily Values are based on a 2,000 calorie diet. Your daily values may be higher or lower depending on your calorie needs:

	Calories	2,000	2,500
Total Fat	Less than	65g	80g
Sat. Fat	Less than	20g	25g
Cholesterol	Less than	300g	300mg
Sodium	Less than	2,400mg	2,400mg
Potassium		3,500mg	3,500mg
Total Carbohydrate		300g	375g
Dietary Fiber		25g	30g
Protein		50g	65g

More Nutrients may be listed on some labels

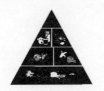

TOTAL FAT
Aim low: Most people need to cut back on fat! Too much fat may contribute to heart disease and cancer. Try to limit your calories from fat. For a healthy heart choose foods with a big difference between the total number of calories and the number of calories from fat.

SATURATED FAT
A new kind of fat? No. Saturated fat is a part of the total fat in food. It is listed separately because it's the key player in raising blood cholesterol and your risk of heart disease. Eat less!

CHOLESTEROL
Too much cholesterol - a second cousin to fat - can lead to heart disease. Challenge yourself to eat less than 300mg each day.

SODIUM
You call it "salt," the label calls it "sodium." Either way, it may add up to high blood pressure in some people. So, keep your sodium intake low-2,400 to 3,000mg or less each day. (The American Heart Association recommends no more than 3,000mg sodium per day for healthy adults.)

DAILY VALUE
Feel like you're drowning in numbers? Let the daily value be your guide. Daily values are listed for people who eat 2,000 or 2,500 calories each day. If you eat more your personal daily value may be higher than what's listed on the label. If you eat less, your personal daily value may be lower. For fat, saturated fat, cholesterol and sodium, choose foods with a low percent daily value. For total carbohydrates, dietary fiber, vitamins and minerals, your daily value goal is to reach 100 percent of each.

g=grams (about 28g = 1 ounce)
mg=milligrams (1,000mg = 1g)
* 7 grams of protein = 1 ounce of protein

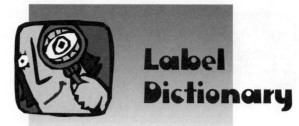

Label Dictionary

Now that you are training yourself to read the labels on the products you purchase from the grocery store, or at least read them before eating anything, you need to know what each item means. This label dictionary will help.

CALORIES	DEFINITION
Light or Lite:	Aside from the USDA established guidelines for whole cuts of meat and poultry, these terms can mean anything - lower in calories, sodium, fat, or even a lighter color!
Low-Calorie:	No more than 40 calories per serving and no more than 0.4 calories per gram of the product.
Reduced-Calorie:	At least one-third fewer calories than the regular item.

Diet or Dietetic: May contain less sodium, cholesterol, calories or a different type of sweetener than in the regular product. Must meet the criteria of either reduced or low-calorie food, or state otherwise.

FAT   DEFINITION

(applies to whole cuts of meat and poultry only)

Light, Lite,   At least 25% less fat than the comparable
Leaner, Lower fat: product.

Lean, Low-fat: At least 90% fat-free by weight.

Extra Lean: At least 95% fat-free by weight.

CHOLESTEROL DEFINITION

Cholesterol-Free: 2 mg. of cholesterol or less per serving.

Low-Cholesterol: 20 mg. of cholesterol or less per serving.

Reduced-Cholesterol: At least a 75% reduction in cholesterol from usual levels.

SWEETENER   DEFINITION

Brown Sugar: White sugar combined with molasses.

Corn Sweeteners,   Syrup or sugar made from corn and corn
Corn Syrup: syrup solids.

Dextrose: A simple sugar also known as glucose.

Fructose: Fruit sugar. Also found in honey.

Glucose: A simple sugar, also known as dextrose.

Granulated Sugar: Crystalline sucrose made from cane or beets.

High-Fructose Corn Syrup (HFCS):	The most commonly used sweetener in processed foods and beverages.
Honey:	A mixture of sucrose, fructose and glucose.
Lactose:	A sugar found in milk and milk products which contains glucose and galactose (a simple sugar). Usually referred to as milk sugar.
Invert Sugar:	A liquid sugar used as a food additive to prevent shrinkage and preserve food freshness.
Maltose:	A sugar which contains two glucose units. Usually referred to as malt sugar.
Mannitol, Sorbitol, Xylitol:	Sugar alcohol, derived from fruits or dextrose.
Maple Sugar and Maple Syrup:	Sugar made from the concentrated sap of the sugar maple tree.
Molasses:	A leftover product of sugar refining.
Sucrose:	Table sugar, beet sugar or cane sugar.
Turbinado sugar:	Raw sugar which has been processed to remove dirt, debris, etc.

SALT	**DEFINITION**
Sodium-Free:	Less than 5 mg. of sodium per serving.
Very Low Sodium:	35 mg. of sodium or less per serving.
Low Sodium:	140 mg. of sodium or less per serving.
Reduced-Sodium:	At least a 75% reduction in sodium from the usual levels.

| Unsalted, Without Added Salt, No Salt Added and Salt Free: | No salt added during processing (to a food normally processed with salt). The items may still contain sodium from other ingredients such as baking soda (e.g. sodium bicarbonate). |

SUGAR	**DEFINITION**
Sugar-Free Sugarless, No Sugar:	This product is not sweetened with sucrose, corn syrup, honey or fructose. It may contain other sweeteners like sugar alcohol such as sorbitol, mannitol or xylitol that do contain calories.
No Sugar Added:	The product contains no "sugar" but may be sweetened with concentrated fruit juices. Keep in mind that these sweeteners do add calories.

GENERAL	**DEFINITION**
No Preservatives:	Can be misleading because the product may have other additives such as artificial colors, flavors or emulsifiers.
Organic Food:	Has no legal definition according to the FDA. But it has a popular definition that is legal in certain states: A food or nutrient that has been produced without the use of chemical fertilizers, pesticides or additives.
New:	Cannot stay on a label for more than six months.

Natural: The USDA has established guidelines for
                  meat and poultry only. For meat and
                  poultry it means that the food item has
                  been minimally processed and contains no
                  artificial ingredients or preservatives. The
                  Council of Better Business Bureaus has
                  loosely interpreted "natural" to include ice
                  cream, carbonated beverages, chewing gum,
                  syrup, flavored drink mixes, pan spray
                  coating and purified fructose.

Health Food: Has no legal definition according to the
                  FDA.

High Fiber: A food containing any amount of fiber can
                  use this term. No regulations for using this
                  term have been established.

chapter sixteen

Get a Grip When You Party

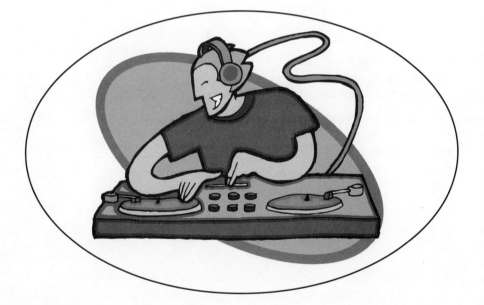

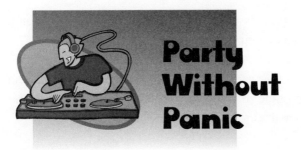

Party Without Panic

If it's "Party Time," it's time to celebrate, not panic! Just because there may be food around doesn't mean you need to freak out because you think you can't control your eating. OF COURSE YOU CAN! My "Party Without Panic" tips can be used for any hang-out or vacation time. Make these helpful hints part of your daily life and fill your emotional files full with this information. Never fear... just stop for a moment and think. Since you have now programmed yourself for success, you will automatically make the right decisions!

1. To begin, be sure and drink at least 64 ounces of water every day. This will not only help to flush out the additional fats you may be eating, it will also keep your body hydrated and less thirsty for sodas and high-sugar drinks.

2. Pile up your plate with protein-rich foods like chicken, turkey, and lean meats first. Eat fruits and vegetables whenever possible and try to avoid salads containing heavy mayonnaise or dressings.

3. Sample the desserts. If you like sweets, nibble on a bunch of them instead of eating an entire serving of each one.

4. Never go to a party hungry. Eat a good lunch or protein-rich snack before party time so you're not so hungry that you binge on high calorie chips, dips and hors d'oeuvres.

5. Eat treats only when you go out. If you know you're going to a lot of parties over the weekend, stay away from any food that isn't really great for you when you're home. Save your 'junk food' time for special events.

6. You can't live on party food. Try and keep meals as lean and well balanced as possible and eat properly at every opportunity.

7. Eat grilled or broiled items from both fast food and restaurant menus.

8. Keep quick snacks like low-fat yogurt, fresh fruit, meat chunks and raw vegetables handy and pre-cut in your refrigerator so you can eat them between events. Healthy snacks need to be readily available and easy to be eaten. We don't tend to take the time to prepare foods that are good for us - it's easier to grab a handful of chips.

9. Don't keep cookies, cakes or chips at home. If you're the host of the party, send the remaining party foods home with your guests. Make it inconvenient to eat things you know you should try and stay away from.

10. If you must eat in fast food restaurants, be a fast food expert. Find places that make things you like that are good for you and be aware of the healthy options you can have at the places you go to most.

11. If your friends are going for pizza, fill up on a salad first so you eat fewer pizza slices and less of the carbs and cheese.

12. If you're going to the movies, drink water instead of soda and don't put the "buttery topping" on the popcorn. The stuff they use as 'butter' is usually some kind of flavored oil that is full of fat and chemicals. Stay away from it!

13. Bring your own snack. If you're going somewhere that snack items are all that's being served, carry a high-protein nutrition bar with you and eat that instead. There are great chocolate covered protein bars available that have 15-20 grams of protein with very low carbohydrate counts. Read the label to be sure you're not buying a body-building carbohydrate-enriched bar. Keep high-protein, low-carb bars handy. They will help you avoid the temptation to eat regular candy bars, and will fill you up in the process.

14. Anytime you feel full and are not hungry....DON'T EAT! We sometimes tend to eat food just because it's there and not because we're hungry. Break this habit. If the party gets boring, leave! Don't just hang around and eat a bunch of junk you don't want because you don't have anything better to do.

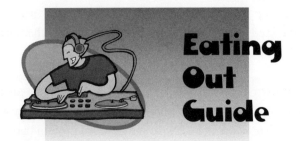

Eating Out Guide

Going out to eat should be fun, not scary or depressing. Now that you know how to eat, picking food that's good for your body is a snap. Even though you may want to plan your food for the day if you know you're going out, I don't want you to starve yourself and eat nothing just to get ready to eat tonight! Starving yourself is the worst thing you could do because, when you're overly hungry, you will tend to eat more. If you find yourself starving by the time the dinner rolls come around, you can be sure you will eat much more bread than you would if you were not so hungry.

When you know where you will be having dinner, just plan the rest of your meals for that day around what you think you'll pick as your dinner entrée. If you know you're eating Italian food and pasta is going to be your likely choice, then "bag" the bread or cereal for breakfast and lunch.

Your metabolism must be active throughout the day in order to maintain an elevated level to help you lose weight. When you don't eat, you are slowing your metabolism while you're making yourself really hungry. Think about it. Slow metabolism and extreme hunger...what a bad combination!

Since dining out should be a wonderful and stress-free experience, this is what you can do:

Be Selective About Restaurants. Whenever possible, you pick the restaurant that you like to go to the most. Find one that offers the kind of food you like best. When someone else is choosing the restaurant, and you are unsure of the type of food they serve, you can always call ahead and ask what is on their menu. Big chain restaurants like Fridays, Fuddrucker's, Denny's, Outback, Bobby Rabino's, Tony Roma's, or Pizza Hut, all offer anything from burgers and pizza, to steak. Try to avoid fast-food restaurants whenever you can. Your healthy food options are very limited there.

When you're checking out the menu, if every option you see seems full of excess calories because of sauces or cheese, simply ask if the chef can make you something lighter or ask them to keep the fatty sauces off the meal or serve them on the side. It is very unusual for any restaurant not to offer some type of grilled entrée like steak, chicken dishes, or seafood.

Make It Worth It. When I am thinking about eating something that I know I should probably stay away from, I simply ask myself if this food is "worth it." "Worth it" foods are those that are very high in fat or calories, but taste so good! You can't eat these things all the time. But, if you are going to eat something you know is not really good for you, at least be sure it's "worth it." Bread and desserts are always good examples of "worth it" foods. Don't eat bread just because it's sitting in front of you. If the rolls look really amazing - hot, fresh and seasoned, then go for it. If not, pass. The same rule holds true for desserts. If you order something and it is not as wonderful as you thought it would be, stop eating it. There is no reason to feel guilty about eating something you know you shouldn't if the experience is not "worth it!"

If plain ol' bread is too great a temptation to have sitting on the table, have the waiter take it away! You can even take one piece if you want, then ask the waiter to remove the rest. Don't sit with something you'd love to eat, staring you in the face. There is nothing wrong with being weak on willpower. Just recognize your weakness and take away anything you'd prefer to stay away from.

When In Doubt....Ask! When eating out, remember that you are the customer. If there is something you don't understand about any menu item or want to know how something is prepared, ask the waiter. Be sure that you are fully aware of what you ordered and that the meal you chose falls within your eating guidelines. Questions like: "Is it fried?", "Is it broiled?", "Does this come with a sauce on top?" should become part of your ordering process for the rest of your life.

Keep Sauces On The Side. Sauces and salad dressings can double or triple the fat content of a meal. Some people only want the taste of sauces or dressings and are happy to dip into a side plate rather than pour the sauce all over the food. To be safe, you can always ask for any high-fat item like butter, sour cream, dressings and sauces to be served "on the side" so you can control how much of it you eat.

Don't Over-eat, Just Take It Home. Even though Mom taught you to clean your plate...don't do it. Whatever you are eating tonight will be just about as good tomorrow. When you are full, stop eating and take home the leftovers.

'Sharing' Is Not A Dirty Word. If you are not very hungry, order a light appetizer like soup or salad for yourself and share an entreé with your friend or dining companion. You may also want to order a separate vegetable or side dish to go along with the main course. Sharing is an especially good idea if you would like to have dessert after the meal. When you share, you get the benefit of tasting the items you like without feeling like you have to finish all the food by yourself.

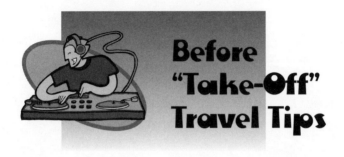

Before "Take-Off" Travel Tips

If you fly a lot or even if you only take the occasional airplane ride, you will still be exposed to the unhealthy effects of flying. You will be getting ready for your trip so take a few minutes to get ready for your flight, too. It is amazing how a few simple tips can help you avoid getting jet-sick and jet-lagged.

Airplanes are a hot bed for germs. The person sitting in row 46 will personally experience the sneeze made by the passenger in row 8. Since most jets provide only 40% to 60% fresh air, the rest is recirculated through a filter system that generally does not remove germs. That means that the germs that are flying around in the cabin air continue to go back and forth between passengers. As if this isn't bad enough, cabin air is not only recycled, it is incredibly dry. The humidity level of cabin air is often only 20% and sometimes dips as low as zero. If you're not sure what these percentages mean, the air in the plane is usually drier than most desert air that contains at least 15-20% humidity!

Since the extremely dry airplane environment will cause the protective mucus layers in your nose, mouth, and throat to dry out, you could find yourself with a microbian infection, which is basically a cold. To help ward-off the chance of this happening, doctors suggest that you should take two 500 milligram capsules of echinacea, 1000-2000 milligrams of vitamin C and 25,000 units of beta-carotene a day before you leave on your trip, then repeat this dosage again a few hours before departure as well.

Bring your own water bottle on the plane and drink as much as you can. The lack of humidity in the plane's air can cause dehydration, fatigue, dry skin, dry and itchy eyes, light-headedness and headache, so, drink lots of water - preferably non-carbonated water. Doctors recommend between 12-16 ounces PER HOUR. It is best if you bring bottled water with you since it is not always easy to get quality water on the plane. And, don't forget, if you use a water bottle that has a straw or sports cap, you will be able to drink two to three times more.

Don't drink caffeinated beverages like colas or coffee during your flight. Both act as diuretics that make your body lose water and can further agitate dehydration.

Since the food served on airplanes is either gross, inedible, nutritionally unsound or non-existent, I suggest either eating before your flight or taking healthy food along with you. Fruit packs pretty well and you can also bring a sandwich made from low-fat protein. Keeping your stomach full is more comforting and it also lessens the possibility of getting airsick.

All of this may seem overwhelming, but it's not. A little planning goes a long way to ensure your comfort and safety. It's no fun landing somewhere only to find yourself sick and in bed for the rest of your vacation. Even though you are sure none of these possible conditions will happen to you, why not be safe rather than sorry?

chapter seventeen

Puking Isn't Sexy

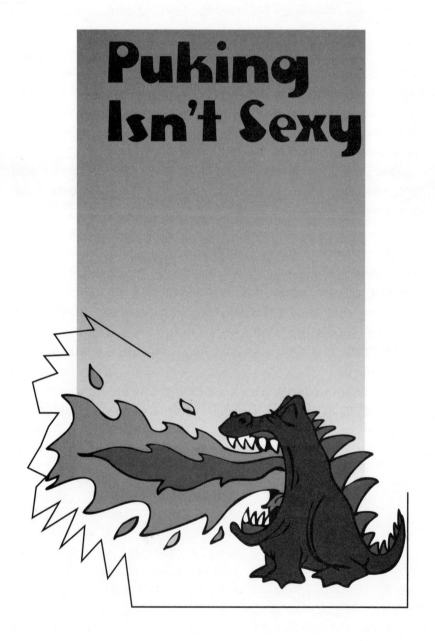

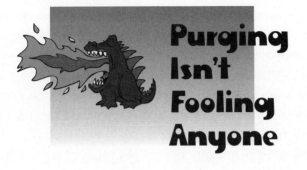

Purging Isn't Fooling Anyone

I am always surprised by how acceptable many teens feel that it is to simply throw up after a meal and remove all the over-indulgences from their bodies. This is a practice that is not only done at home, it's also done when they are out with friends. Sometimes the friends know. Sometimes they don't. But, most often the person throwing up thinks that they have fooled everyone.

Anxiety and upset aren't things that you can make go away simply by using willpower. If this chapter pertains to you or someone you love, read it carefully. Anorexia and bulimia are the result of false beliefs. You are convinced that you can best control yourself by failing to eat, or eating then purging yourself of the 'mistake.' But, food isn't your enemy. Food didn't do anything to you but try and nourish your body. The enemy is the condition or situation that you would rather not face. And, while you run away from it, you are only making yourself sicker and more unhappy.

When people who love you and care about you know that you are vomiting after meals, they don't always say anything because they feel helpless. Many parents think this is just a temporary phase or a "teenage thing" that you will miraculously grow out of. They want to believe that whatever is bothering you, will just go away. Unfortunately, it won't.

Nothing is going away until you tell it to. And, you can't tell yourself anything that you are unwilling to face.

When people don't understand you, you feel even more isolated. If your situation makes no sense to them because they just don't 'get it,' then you feel frustrated. Isolation and frustration can show up in a lot of different ways... attitude... drug use... alcohol... food.

A problem is just a problem. It doesn't have to be any bigger or any smaller than we allow it to be. If we take a little thing like a fight with a friend and turn it into what seems like the end of the world, it will be a problem. Remember, your reality IS what you believe it is. Always keep in mind that a belief is just a belief until you change your mind and decide to believe something else.

If you think you can control your body, your weight and how you look by just purging yourself of the food you eat, then that is your belief. It doesn't make it true, it just makes it 'real' for you. The people around you know that you aren't in control but you have successfully fooled yourself into thinking that you are. I could honestly believe that I could fly, but that doesn't make it true to anyone other than me.

Now is the time to let the logical side of your brain work for a minute. The emotional side has been controlling your actions up until now and telling you that it is all right to purge yourself when you overeat. You have created an entire filing cabinet of emotional belief files that support and justify that decision. But, your logical side knows better. You just need to listen to what it has to say, and make the decision to clean out the emotional files that are no longer of use to you now. Let's take a look at a few logical facts that I'm sure you'll agree with:

- Your body needs food to live.
- You can't be healthy if you deny your body nutrition.
- You can't feel good if your body is empty.
- Weight control means creating good eating habits.
- Lifetime weight maintenance means consistent and manageable food behaviors.
- You are no happier after purging than you were before purging.

Logically, you recognize that you have not selected the best option for weight control if you have been using bulimia as your program. You are not alone in these activities. Studies have shown that by the first year of college, up to 18% of women and 4% of men have had a history of bulimia. Approximately the same percentages hold true for anorexia.

This is a life-threatening disease that kills thousands every year. The profile of these individuals shows:

- Low self-esteem
- Compulsive behaviors
- Tend to over-exercise
- Achievers
- Regularly depressed
- Push food around on their plate
- Eat secretively

Purging affects the body's balance of sodium, potassium, and other chemicals. It causes fatigue, thinner bones, irregular heartbeat and even seizures. Constant vomiting can damage the stomach and esophagus, cause irregular menstrual cycles, create broken blood vessels in the face, skin rashes, erode tooth enamel, and make the gums recede.

If you or someone you know is bulimic, this is the reality check of what you or your friends are doing to yourselves. This is the real reality, not the emotionally believed one. If your appearance is that important to you, do you really want to look the way you will end up looking if you continue to abuse yourself?

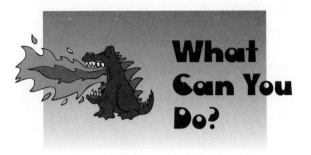

What Can You Do?

If you want to know what you can do when you have an eating disorder, first and foremost - FACE IT. Tell your friends and family that you have a problem and don't be surprised if they already know. Ask for their help and let them give it to you.

Most people handle bulimia or anorexia therapy best if they get professional help. Before you start, you can take a look through your emotional files and see what is drawing you to this behavior. Why do you believe that purging is your solution to weight management?

Take each one of the items listed in the profile and list all the reasons why that item applies to you.

• **Low self-esteem:**
    Am I jealous of others?
    Do I think I am inferior?
    Do I think I am untalented?
    Am I not as pretty or thin as others?
    Am I not as smart?
    Do others have nicer possessions?
    What do I think I am lacking that others have?

• **Compulsive behaviors:**

How important are drugs or alcohol to me?
When I start something, is it difficult to stop?
Do I act without thinking?
Can I be counted on?

• **Achievers:**

Am I a perfectionist?
Do I feel I must always be the best?
How do I respond when I don't do as well as I would like?
Do my parents or teachers have unrealistic expectations?
Why do I feel I am driven to succeed?

• **Regularly depressed:**

Am I unhappy more than I am happy?
What makes me unhappy?
    Friends?
    Family?
    Relationships?
    School?
    Pressures?
    Appearance?
    Fitting in?

• **Why?**

Why do I purge myself?
How do I feel afterward? Better? Worse?
What problems do I think my purging solved?
What goal does this behavior promote?

As you do this exercise, you will begin to create a new picture of yourself. This should be done without emotions. The logical side of your brain is now in control. You are merely looking at your emotional responses to conditions, you are not reliving them. When you understand what you do or how you react to different challenges that you must deal with, you can make changes that will make you happier.

Changing emotional responses isn't always easy, that's why professional help can guide you and make the transition easier. Don't be afraid of opening up and learning everything you can about yourself. Every problem and conflict you solve now is just one less that you will need to face later. And, the sooner these conflicts are faced, the sooner the stress associated with them can be eliminated.

chapter eighteen

Unorganized Exercise

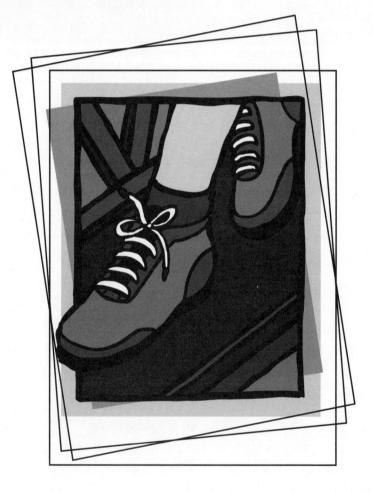

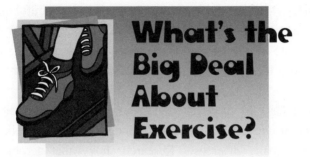

What's the Big Deal About Exercise?

Are you a couch potato? National statistics show that kids show less interest in exercise than ever before. Most spend their extra free time on the internet, the phone or watching TV. Even physical education in school is a thing of the past, unless you're participating in one of the organized sport activities. Even though all this is true, we still always feel better when we show some physical exertion. And, best of all, exercise doesn't have to be painful or difficult in order to be effective...it can even be fun. You can turn your body into a calorie-burner instead of a calorie-saver with exercise.

Just to keep you up-to-speed on the "whys" of your potential new activities, let me tell you that aerobic activities benefit your heart. The word 'aerobic' literally means with oxygen. When you do aerobic exercise, your goal is to keep your heart rate up over a given period of time. Initially, you may not be able to keep your heart rate at a higher level for very long. Start slowly, and build up. As you begin to exercise more often, you will be surprised at how much more exercise you'll be able to do.

Weight training focuses more on muscle development than the heart. This is also a good option for those who prefer not to 'sweat' as much. Using weights will help you reshape your body, increase lean muscle and bone mass, while making you stronger.

If you haven't done much exercise before now, be careful not to over-train in your enthusiasm. Let your muscles rest every other day until you feel you can do more. And, if the exercise you pick requires some physical endurance like running or biking, be sure to stretch-out before you begin.

Exercise has a lot more than the obvious benefits. In addition to the calorie and fat-burning that exercise offers, it is also an excellent way to help prevent many diseases. Research shows that aerobic exercise reduces joint pain and arthritis symptoms. Exercise also helps with osteoporosis, hypertension, premenstrual symptoms and helps keep blood sugar levels in a normal range for diabetics. Cholesterol levels are also reduced with cardiovascular stimulation.

Additional benefits include:

- You'll look better
- You'll feel better
- You'll have more energy
- Exercise relieves stress
- It burns up lots of calories
- It increases your mind's ability to focus
- And, it feels great when you're done!

Although it's important that you exercise whenever you can, cramming in your workout whenever it fits into your schedule may not be as beneficial as it would if you took your time. The time of day can play an important role in making the most of your exercise efforts, too. Studies show that pain-tolerance is higher before noon so, if you have a mild injury or your muscles are sore, plan your workout for the morning.

- Muscle strength tends to peak between noon and 6:00 PM making afternoons the best time for weight lifting.

• Hand-eye coordination, manual dexterity and reaction time all peak between 2:30 PM and 4:00 PM - prime time for sports like tennis.

• Muscles warm up as the day goes along, so stretch related workouts like yoga or gymnastics are best during early evening.

• For many sports, performance improves as the day progresses. Swimmers, for instance, hit their peak speed around 10:00 in the evening.

With a little planning, your workout and your exercise performance can be more productive and effective.   Any exercise is better than no exercise at all. Even walking one day a week will begin to get you programmed to walk more often. You'll be amazed at how quickly your body will respond and crave more!

Exercise is not about how long you do it, it's about the quality of your activity. Quite honestly, too much exercise can be just as ineffective as not enough. Short and intense workouts produce the best results while helping you to relieve stress and get your mind ready for a more productive day. Anytime you do something that is so good for you but doesn't come naturally, you're making great strides in taking control of YOU.

Exercise can also be a great family experience. Ask a parent, brother or sister to workout with you. This becomes a great bonding time, especially if you have little in common with your workout buddy otherwise. Both my children workout with their dad several times a week and have gone from hating exercise to looking forward to their gym time with him. That's one activity where they all get along!

A healthy vision requires physical fitness. Make exercise an automatic part of your life. Be good to yourself and let a little exercise help create a better balance for you day-to-day. If you currently do not do much exercise, identify all of the benefits exercise will provide for you and picture yourself exercising regularly. Fill your emotional filing cabinet with positive feelings about exercise until your current, negative feelings have been replaced. Your body and your lifestyle will thank you for it!

HOW EXERCISE WORKS FOR WEIGHT LOSS

We already know that losing unwanted fat is your goal. Why exercise? Simple. You can eat more when you keep muscle and lose fat! When you change what you're eating to lower calories and you don't exercise, you are losing some fat but you are also loosing muscle mass at the same time. 25% of all weight lost without exercise comes from muscle loss which isn't good. Muscle burns 40 calories per pound. Fat burns 2 calories per pound. You do the math!!!

What does all this mean to you? Simple. Get rid of the fat and build up the muscle. The heavier you are or the higher your body fat content, the fewer calories you can eat every day just to stay the same size that you are now. My job is to help show you how to lose more fat without losing muscle. Or, better yet, build up your muscle mass so you will be able to eat more and still be thinner. Pretty cool, huh?

You don't have to exercise every day or kill yourself doing exercise either in order to build your muscles up. Surprisingly enough, the good news is that "less is more" when it comes to exercising for weight loss.

YOU HAVE TWO OPTIONS:

Aerobic exercises, which are heart elevating exercises like running, biking, tennis, basketball, volleyball and soccer, all burn fat. To get the most out of your aerobic workout, all you need to do is get your heart rate up just a little above normal and keep it there for 20 minutes and you will burn the maximum amount of fat possible.

To calculate the best weight loss heart range for you, all you need to do is deduct your age from 220 then take 70-80% of that number. Here's how to do it:

If you are 15 years old: 220 - 15 = 205
70% of 205 = 143 / 80% of 205 = 164

To burn as much fat as a 15 year old can, you'll need to keep your heart rate between 143 and 164 beats per minute for 20 minutes straight while you are exercising. Getting your heart to go up to those levels is much easier than you may think. In fact, you may not even break a sweat, but your exercise effort will still burn the fat. Experts tell us that if you get your heart rate up too high, (following the "no pain /no gain" concept) it will not work anymore when it comes to fat burn and weight management. You need to keep your heart in the right range for your age when you do aerobic exercises so your body can use your fat storage for energy.

Anaerobic exercises are resistance or weight training exercises that are designed to burn up the sugar your body creates eating sweets or starches. This kind of training actually burns the sugar while it is building muscle. Weight training exercises makes the body burn glucose or sugar for energy, not fat. But, by maintaining or building up your muscle mass while you are trying to lose weight, your body is able to process more calories through it's systems so you can eat more. Remember, muscle burns 40 calories per pound and fat burns only 2 calories per pound. The more muscles you have, the more you can eat.

Over-exercising or getting your heart beat up too high when you are doing aerobic exercises is not good. You will actually put your body into what is called an "anaerobic state". That means you have reached a place where your body stops burning fat and starts building muscle instead. Building muscle is good once you have reached your goal weight but it is not good when you are over-exercising and stopping the fat from burning up. Once your heart gets higher than the top of the 80% level we did for your age, you can't just slow down and let your body start over. You actually have to stop exercising for at least one hour later or come back on another day and start again.

Heart Monitors help you get it right because they allow you to know by the little clock-like dial that you are keeping your heart rate within your personal fat-burning range. Heart rate monitors work for your body like a tachometer works in a car. It shows you how hard your engine is working. You can get heart monitors at drug or department stores. They are easy to wear too. You just Velcro the strap around your chest and wear the watch that goes with it. It is very simple to use and the instructions will come in the box for the specific model that you buy.

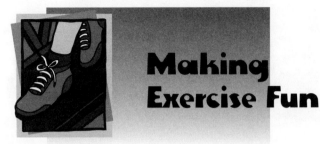

Making Exercise Fun

You don't have to exercise in order to lose weight, but it's logical that any activities you do pretty often will help increase your heart rate and elevate your metabolism. This will ultimately increase your weight loss success, too. Many people don't mind exercise as long as they don't have to sweat or do aerobics. In fact, isometric exercise which involves contracting muscles against high resistance, like weights, is actually more effective for losing weight. It builds muscle mass while helping to firm and tone the body.

Expensive trainers or equipment are not needed if you have the desire to firm-up. Working your body against itself can be very effective and you can also use stuff you have around the house like brooms or water bottles to add extra stretch or weight.

Be creative and enjoy exercising. Make it a family affair and invite mom, dad, a sibling or a friend to join you. Play outdoor games or roughhouse with the dog. Whatever you do to help elevate your heart is a form of exercise. Check out the mini-workouts section of this book for a few silly, fun and effective exercise suggestions. It's time to get off the couch, get your butt in gear and MOVE!

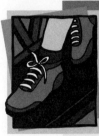

Mini-Workouts May Be All You Need

With your days packed full of school, friends, family and other stuff, I know it can be tough to squeeze exercise into your schedule. Well, you'll be happy to know that shorter workouts a couple of times each day were proven to be just as effective as one, long exercise program.

People who break their exercise into 4 ten-minute workouts daily do a much better job and enjoy their exercise more than people who try to tackle their daily exercise all in one shot. According to one study, people who try to take forty-five minutes to an hour each day to exercise got tired of their exercise program, found the time requirement too hard to keep up, and stopped working out altogether in a relatively short period of time. The other group that only did 10-minute workouts four times a day didn't mind the break in their regular routine and continued to exercise after the study was over.

If you're not a big fan of traditional exercise and don't have the time or money needed to join a gym, here are a few activities you can try that will strengthen your heart and burn a few extra calories:

Walk Your Dog: Not only will this exercise give you a practical way to raise your heart rate with some aerobic stimulation, it gives you time to bond with a loving friend.

Park Far Away When Shopping: Walking is always good exercise. When you park away from your shopping destination, you will get extra exercise just going to the store. And, should you actually buy something, you will have the opportunity to strengthen your arms even more by carrying your new items back to the car!

Take Extra Trips On Your Staircase: Don't put everything that needs to go upstairs on the bottom step, take the items up the stairs as you collect them. If your room is downstairs, help mom out. You may even want to take a few extra trips up and down your staircase just for the 'heart' of it.

In The Pool, Tread Water: Great cardiovascular exercise.

Use Swim Fins: Kick in the water holding onto the side. This is a great exercise to help increase the circulation in your feet and legs and, it can even be done in the bathtub.

Aquatic Jogging: Run in place or back & forth across the shallow end of the pool. The water resistance is great for your legs.

Volleyball: Fun for the whole family and great preparation for the next olympic games!

Step Up: Try step aerobics on two steps in the pool or in your house. Keep with the beat of your favorite radio station or CD and have fun.

Sports Challenge: Play basketball, tennis or other sports with a friend.

Hold The Handles: Use 2 large, empty bleach containers and try to get them to touch underwater...great for your arms and shoulders. You can even carry two full bleach containers around the house with you - that will give your arms a workout, too.

Lift & Stretch: Stand holding the side of a door and lift each leg out one at a time. This is great to help tighten your buttocks.

Resistance Weights & Boots. Available for land or water use and helps increase the value of your exercise.

Bicycle: This is a non-weight bearing exercise that can save on gas money, encourage your appreciation of your local surroundings and still promote aerobic activity.

Sit Up Straight: If you 'slump' it is amazing how much you can strengthen your back by sitting up straight at home or school.

Skate: Rollerblading is a great form of transportation and great for your heart and legs.

Sit Ups: With feet elevated through the footboard of a bed, tighten up the stomach and back of the legs.

Circular Arm Rotations: Six to eight inches in diameter, first back then forward, tightens up the flabbiness under the arms. Doing this exercise while holding a large full can or bleach bottle in each hand will add additional pressure.

Use A Broomstick: Placing a broomstick across your back and under each arm while stretching side to side will trim down the waist.

Pelvic Tilts. Put a phone book or two on your tummy, this will burn bulges off your butt.

Weight Loss Is The Best Exercise Of All!

Exercise is important. But, just losing weight is the best solution for your overall health. It is important that you stay active. Active people not only have more productive lives, they live longer. If organized exercise does not appeal to you, find options that do, but get your weight under control first.

chapter nineteen

Smoking & Weight Management

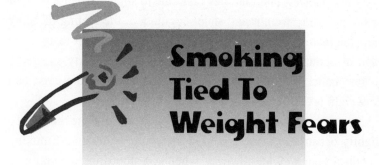

Smoking Tied To Weight Fears

If you think smoking will keep you from eating, think again. There is no question that many young people smoke because they think it will prevent weight gain, but the only thing anybody is going to lose just by smoking is their good health.

Cigarettes don't prevent weight gain and they certainly don't promote weight loss. Cigarettes don't suppress your appetite so if you tend to overeat when you don't smoke, you will still tend to overeat if you do smoke. Many people, young and old, believe that because you put cigarettes in your mouth, this action will replace putting food in your mouth instead. This belief also gives a false reason for a habit that is not only bad for you, it is banned from most public establishments like restaurants, movie theaters and stores. No studies have ever confirmed that smoking assists weight management, so get that thought out of your head.

If you smoke because you think it will help you with your weight, you're incorrect but not alone in your thinking. When conducting a study with 10-17 year olds, researchers found that more than 30% of the young people they interviewed said that they continue to smoke because of their "anxieties about body weight and shape regulation, the feeling of being too fat, and the fear of losing control of eating." Young adults that gained an average of about 15 pounds in their weight since puberty showed a 70% greater chance of smoking in order to maintain a more even and desirable weight level.

Smoking has no effect on your appetite, but it will elevate the metabolism slightly because nicotine is a mild metabolic stimulant. Smoking will not control your weight, however, when you stop smoking, you may possibly experience a small weight gain. Your gain is not because you would start to eat more, but because your metabolism will slow at this weight level from the lack of nicotine in your system.

The physical health dangers associated with smoking are a lot worse than any of the wrongly assumed weight management benefits. Since most smokers smoke every day, their body will get used to the metabolic stimulation from the number of cigarettes they usually smoke. If you are overweight and smoke, (most people smoke about the same number of cigarettes every day) your body is used to smoking a given number of cigarettes to maintain its current size. This metabolic condition is just like exercise. If you are overweight and you currently jog three times per week for 1 mile each day, your body will stay overweight until you do additional exercise, like 2 miles each day, to stimulate your metabolism further.

You are much better off regulating your eating and using exercise to help elevate your metabolism rather than try and stimulate it through smoking. Since there are no appetite control properties to cigarettes, and long-term smoking can eventually kill you, a healthier option makes more sense. You still need to take control of the food you eat and learn to make smart choices. Cigarettes will not assist you in any of these efforts so don't use smoking as a weight-control excuse anymore.

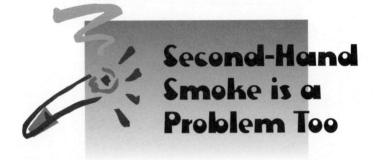

Second-Hand Smoke is a Problem Too

I find it amazing that even with so much information given to us on the dangers of smoking, there are still so many households that contain smokers. The statistics can be staggering: Almost 23% of American women smoke cigarettes.

Each year, smoking causes more deaths in the United States than AIDS, alcohol, automobile accidents, fires, homicides, illicit drugs and suicide COMBINED!!! And still some people choose to smoke. Are they nuts or what???

For women, lung cancer is the number one cause of cancer related death. And, women who take birth control pills and smoke increase their risk of stroke and heart attack even more.

What is even sadder is that smoking is affecting those non-smokers who are forced to live with or be around smokers. Parents who smoke make breathing really hard for family members who are prone to bronchitis, asthma, and ear infections. Passive smoke may also increase kids' risk of lung disease as adults. Regular exposure to smoke puts kids at a greater risk for early heart disease, too.

A study conducted showed that kids living in homes with parents who smoke had a 10% less protective HDL (good) cholesterol level than those living with non-smoking parents. Even children of light smokers suffered negative effects. Since kids rarely have cholesterol problems, researchers evaluated those with inherited high cholesterol. But the findings may point to long-term heart troubles for all kids whose parents smoke, including those with normal cholesterol levels during childhood.

If your parents smoke, encourage them to quit. They will be doing themselves and their loved ones a favor. You are going through a lot of changes to improve your health and your body. Your parents can show the same drive and initiative, so encourage them to do something that will greatly improve the health of the entire family, not to mention the length of their own life.

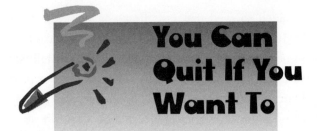

You Can Quit If You Want To

If you want to quit smoking, you can. By using my visualization process, you can do a reverse of the positive images you are creating about weight loss and start to program negative images in association with the activity of smoking. But, just like with weight loss, you need to first identify the negative images that would most motivate you to quit.

Make a list of all the reasons you can think of why you would want to stop smoking. Here are a few suggestions to get you started, but I'm sure you'll have a few more of your own to include:

- Your clothes smell of smoke and people avoid you.
- Your hair smells like cigarettes.
- Your boyfriend or girlfriend doesn't want to kiss you because you taste like cigarettes.
- You will get wrinkled and age badly from smoking.
- Your fingers and nails become stained and ugly.
- The people you love get cancer from YOUR second-hand smoke.
- You can die of lung cancer.

- Friends don't want to let you in their car because you stink.
- People don't want to date you because you are a "smoker."
- Your brother or sister looks up to you and you are a bad example for them now.
- It upsets your family that you smoke.
- People you have not yet met have the wrong impression of who you are because you smoke.
- Your teeth become yellow and gross.
- You get gum disease.
- The walls of the room where you smoke become discolored from nicotine stains.
- You find it hard to breathe.
- You can't keep up with everyone else in gym because you are constantly out of breath.
- You develop an embarrassing cough.
- You spend money on cigarettes that could be better spent on other things.
- You eat more because your food is tasteless.
- You get sick really often.

Now, when you visualize a thinner, healthier and more vibrant YOU, you will also think about why smoking is no longer a part of that image because of all the reasons you have listed. Your visions will be of people turning away from you because of your smoking. This will make the act of smoking a negative one that needs to be removed from your emotional support files.

You already know there is no "good reason" for smoking. Eventually, you will need to quit anyway and the sooner you decide to do that, the healthier you and the people around you will be.

chapter twenty

Putting The Program All Together

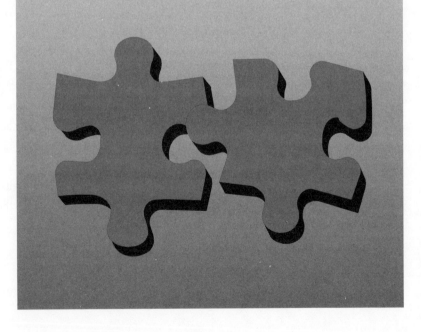

Let's Put it All Together

You're almost there! When you have a clear picture of the goals you want to achieve, you can map out the path you are willing to take in order to achieve them. The path must be yours, not the direction of someone else. Only you can look at yourself and know how you want to live your life...how you want to look and feel. These are your decisions, and yours alone. Nobody can want more for you than you want for yourself. You have the ability within yourself to accomplish every goal you set. It just takes vision, belief and the willingness to change.

See it...Believe it...Make it happen!

Now that you understand the individual tools you have available to make your weight loss dream a reality, you want to create total balance in your life by blending all aspects of this program together.

Let's recap your direction:

1. Visualize your personal picture. Make a picture in your mind of how you want to look and feel. See it, believe that you can do it, then create a game plan you can live with to make it happen.

2. Plan your picture's reality by writing down, step-by-step, the changes you need to make in your eating and living lifestyles.

3. Be your own best cheerleader by seeing the achievements and successes you will experience each day along the way.

4. Tell your friends and family how they can support and help you to create a healthier body and more happiness for yourself.

5. Understand your eating guidelines and put those guidelines into practice.

6. Take time, every week, to make yourself a priority in some way.

7. Make the commitment to exercise, in some form, on a regular basis.

8. Find a weekly project that you can do to improve your health or home life.

9. Feel strong and smart knowing that you have the power inside yourself to visualize your dreams and make those dreams come true.

10. Believe in yourself. You can move mountains... The power is in YOU!

Debi Davis
401 Fairway Drive, Deerfield Beach, FL 33441
www.BioDietetics.com

My Dear Teen,

You should be so proud of yourself. Seeking solutions to difficult problems takes a lot of courage. So does accepting the responsibility for your own actions. You would be surprised at the number of adults that have failed to learn this lesson.

When you chart a course for your life, whether to lose weight or to reach any other goal you may have, you will begin to see that achieving each and every goal is only a matter of planning. When you think about what you need to do to achieve your dreams, and actually plan the strategy for them, you will be surprised at how quickly your life takes on a new and exciting direction.

You will find that behaviors that you no longer find acceptable in yourself will become unacceptable in the people you associate with also. The quality of your relationships will increase. Everything that happens to you and every person that touches your life, plays a role in your personal development. Learn to maximize the positive associations and minimize the negative ones.

Every choice you make is motivated by one of two emotions: Faith or fear. When you believe in yourself and have the faith that you will do your best to make the right decisions in life, you will feel a power and strength within yourself that nobody can ever take from you. Fear makes us justify actions that we know are not in our best interest. Now that you understand that you hold the keys to your own future, you will begin to lock the file drawers that keep you from accomplishing your dreams.

Be confident. Always seek out the information you need to make good, sound decisions. Listen to what people have to say that may know a little more than you. Try out their suggestions. Always keep an open mind.

You have come a long way from the day you first picked up this book. You are now armed with all the information and direction you need to become the person you visualized in your personal picture. Getting this far was the hard part. Losing weight is now a 'piece of cake!'

Please keep in touch and let me know how you're doing along the way. If I can be of any help at all, just write and ask.

Your loving new friend,

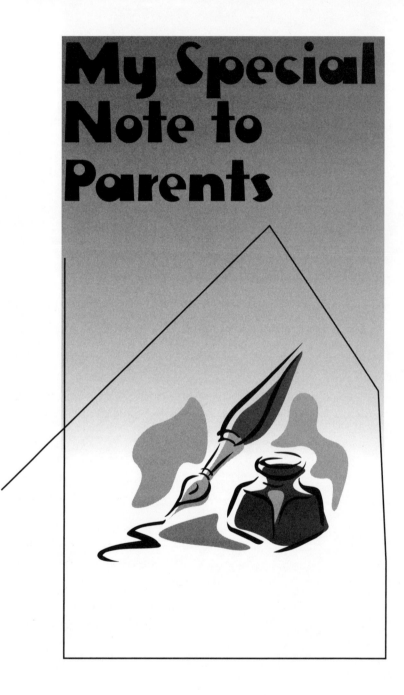

chapter twenty-one

My Special Note to Parents

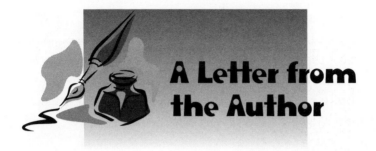

A Letter from the Author

Dear Parents:

I know you're concerned about your child's weight and the way in which they have personally managed their body up until now. Please rest assured that they are just as unhappy and concerned as you are. By reading this book, they are well on their way to finding out how they can reach their ultimate personal goals. With a little of the right information and encouragement, you will be surprised how quickly they will respond. By the end of their reading, they will recognize that a reasonable and easy solution to their problem has been outlined for them. It's now up to them how they use it.

Let them find the way themselves. If they need you, let them reach out. You can certainly make it known that you're available for them, but additional pressure is the last thing they need right now. They've put enough pressure on themselves. Perhaps that's how they got into this predicament in the first place.

Be patient. We all want the best for our children. Empower them by showing that you trust their judgement and let them learn how to want the best for themselves, too. You are a bigger influence on them than you probably realize. Keep the influence positive and support their decision to do this on their own.

I'm a mom too, and I know what I went through with my daughter when she was twelve years old and 26 pounds overweight. Once I backed away and stopped pushing her to improve her eating and appearance, she made the decision all by herself. Your child will too.

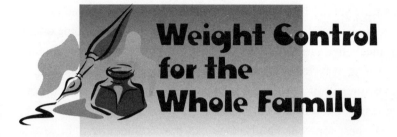

Weight Control for the Whole Family

At least one out of every four children in America is overweight. It is typical that a heavy child also has heavy parents. Or, at least they are not generally the only one in the family who is overweight.

If your child is overweight and the rest of your family is either thin or average in size, please don't single out your overweight child. Good eating habits are important for everyone. If you treat a thinner person in your family as someone that should be rewarded with extra food or special desserts, you are sending the wrong message to everyone and could even be creating a future weight problem for your thinner child.

If you have one family member on a 'diet,' you need to have everyone in the family on the same food plan. Don't separate the overweight family member further by serving them something different than everyone else at mealtime. They are more sensitive and aware of their condition than you may even realize. By continually reminding them of their weight and treating it as a problem, you stigmatize them and isolate them further from the family.

Mealtime should be family time. Regular, good tasting and healthy meals should be a part of your family life. Whether eating at home or eating out, meals that are usually at a set time and provide balanced nutrition go a long way to assist weight management efforts. Snacking is oftentimes a result of not knowing when dinner will be served. If your children learn that you will eat between 6:00 and 6:30 pm, or whatever time works best for your family, they can have something light to tide them over when they come home from school. If they're not sure when you plan to eat, they are more likely to fill up on snacks, then eat again when dinnertime rolls around. This creates unbalanced overeating. And, if you're cooking, make sure your food tastes good. Preparation is important, too.

If you have read this book, you already know that high-fat snacks and sweets should be eliminated from your pantry. There are no family members, thin or heavy, that need these items to be readily available. Fruits should be pre-cut and refrigerated for quick snacks. Leave apples and bananas out on the kitchen counter. If anyone in your family is hungry, they will get into the habit of eating smart instead of eating whatever is convenient.

Soda is another item that should be greatly reduced. Nutrition experts say that it is not unusual for children to drink 1000-1500 calories per day in sugary soft drinks and fruit punches. Frankly, doctors tell us that the elimination of just two regular sodas daily will provide a thirty-pound weight loss over the course of twelve months! Water is what they need, especially if you live in a warm climate. Squeeze in a bit of orange, lemon or lime juice, and the flavor may be more to their liking.

If your children are picky about their food, have them make a grocery trip with you and allow them to pick out the items they would like to eat most. Encourage them to try things they haven't eaten before, and take the time to teach them to read labels. When your child has selected their own fruits, vegetables and snack items, they become responsible for what they eat and cannot blame anyone else for being overweight. Learning to take responsibility for one's actions is a lesson from which everyone can benefit.

Food also plays a part in learning disorders and disabilities. Proper nutrition helps children who are hyperactive or are being treated for attention deficit disorders like ADD or ADHD. Sometimes, controlling diet is more effective than medicating a child.

Plan family activities that include physical exercise. Play basketball together. Go swimming. Parents can greatly help inactive children by creating an environment that encourages them to move and not sit and watch TV or play on the computer. As a parent, you need to be a role model. If you come home from work and park yourself on the couch for the evening, don't expect your children to do otherwise. You lead by example. Encourage your child to go outside and play for at least thirty minutes every day after school. This time provides both a mental break and much needed physical activity. It also provides you with a time to bond with your child in a non-threatening or controversial activity. If you're not up to exercise, look into dance, sports or movement classes that your child may enjoy. If nothing else, take a walk together!

Be supportive, not critical. If one child is chastising another because of their size or their eating habits, make them stop. As an overweight person now residing in a thin suit, I know, first-hand, that we place enough pressure and guilt on ourselves, we don't need to be further belittled by others.

Childhood obesity is not a phase. It is not something your child is going to outgrow. Allowing their overweight condition to continue into adulthood doubles your child's risk of heart disease, stroke, colon cancer and makes them 50 times more likely to develop adult-onset diabetes. You need to be educated yourself as to how to handle this situation before you cause more damage.

Here are a few recommendations:

Wait For Clues: Watch for signs of distress in your child. Are they moody, irritable, or loners who avoid sports activities or friends? Speak with their teachers and see if they interact with other children. Do they sit alone at lunch, sport activities, or after-school programs?

Avoid A Preoccupation With Thinness: Many children, especially teens, are faced daily with having perfect bodies. Every music video and all of the teen idols project a perfect body image. That image creates its own pressure. If they see mom or dad constantly making reference to "eating so much that I'll have to go to the gym for an extra day just to work off tonight's dinner," you are sending your child the wrong message. Being a responsible eater is not the same as having a personal preoccupation with food and appearance. If you are constantly asking your children, or if they hear you constantly asking your spouse, "does this dress or pant make me look fat?," you may be creating an ideal that can lead to a variety of eating disorders. Be careful, you are a bigger example in many ways than you may think.

Communicate: Ask questions and listen to their answers. Questions like:

What's bothering you?
How was school today?
Have you made any new friends lately?

These type of questions will help you better understand your child. Be sure you find the right time to talk. Don't try communicating in the middle of your child's favorite TV program. The time that is needed to work things out must be done on their terms and time schedule, not yours.

Reward Their Efforts: If your child has had a great food week, reward them by doing something together that isn't associated with food. Take them to a movie or buy them a CD they've been wanting. Show them your support by illustrating that food isn't the only reward.

Make A Plan Together: Help your child identify what changes they feel need to be made in your family to help support their efforts, and put those plans into action. Don't allow other family members to belittle or sabotage the plan.

Hide The Scale: Don't make pounds the issue. Make smart eating and activity more important. If they are eating better, the scale will take care of itself. If they think you are not concerned about what the scale says, they will be less critical of themselves which will help boost their much needed self-esteem.

Give Unconditional Love: The love you feel for your child is not predicated on how big or how small their body is. Let them know that. If you have other children who do not have a weight problem, your overweight child may feel that you love your other children more. Be careful that praise and care are evenly disbursed. Children at this phase of their life are very sensitive and damage easily.

Please recognize that part of your child's success is based upon your willingness to make changes. Their ability to succeed is far more challenged if you are not part of their solution. You may need to overhaul your family's current lifestyle and make healthy eating and living a priority. Once accomplished, you will find that the rewards for everyone involved are well worth the effort.

MAKE IT HAPPEN

You have now come so far
To reach for your goal
and have set your sights on success.

You can visualize and analyze
So you may be your very best.

Each day brings another new challenge
But never one too great to face.

Taking one step at a time
You will face them head on
With beliefs you don't need to erase.

You're strong and secure
And controlling your fate,
Your spirit is free from all strife.

Move forward assured
That this time you'll succeed
For you've taken control of your life.

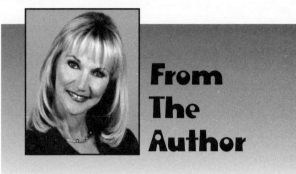

From The Author

The writing of this book comes naturally to me. Having come from an overweight family and personally battling weight problems my entire life, I understand the pain, frustration and depression that being overweight can cause.

In 1991, I was bankrupt, divorced, the mother of two and I was 85 pounds overweight. I had a vision for myself that my physical body and personal lifestyle did not portray. I decided to "live my vision" and lost 85 pounds in less than 6 months which ultimately changed my life.

Following the same strategy that I cover in this book I started losing weight. It did not take long for everyone I was in contact with to ask me what I was doing and inquired if they could do it, too.

Using my watch as collateral to start my company. BioDietetics (formerly Fit America) was born.

Although BioDietetics, which is headquartered in Florida, offers a variety of protein and nutritional supplements, I always remind people to eat regular food, too. Meals are important and learning to eat balanced, healthy and tasty meals will enable you to maintain your new weight forever.

Through this unique visualization process, I am sharing with you the steps I took to regain the power I almost forgot I had. You, and your family, can create the bodies you want by getting back in touch with your mental and physical health.

More than 70% of Americans feel they need to lose weight. When you keep your expectations realistic and your mind occupied with thoughts other than food, you are well on your way to reaching your weight loss goal and a longer, happier, healthier and more rewarding life.

Best wishes to you all.

Acknowledgements

There are so many people that influence the creation of a book. Many doctors and behavioral specialists have helped guide me to a point of understanding that enabled me to translate their wisdom into practicality and share it with others.

I especially want to thank my Fit America/BioDietetics family who support my direction with glowing enthusiasm; Byron, who has been my life-partner in so many ways; Diane Terman- Felenstein, who continues to open doors for me; Ariel Benjamin, who showed me the way to clean out my old and unnecessary "files;" Dr. Ellen Sherman, who is my behavioral advisor; and my children, Blake and Cole, who are always a source of insight, strength and inspiration.

In doing my research for this project, I found a lot of additional medical application for the visualization process which was far too extensive and not necessarily applicable to include in this writing. However, if you desire more information for the healing and medical practicality of visualization, I urge you to read the writings of Andrew Weil, M.D., Deepak Chopra, and, most specifically, Herbert Benson, M.D. I found Dr. Benson's *Timeless Healing...The Power and Biology of Belief* to be an invaluable source of information and motivation.